Re

OXFORD MEDICAL PUBLICATI

Research Methods for General Practitioners

Oxford University Press, Walton Street, Oxford OX2 6DP
Oxford   New York   Toronto
Delhi   Bombay   Calcutta   Madras   Karachi
Petaling Jaya   Singapore   Hong Kong   Tokyo
Nairobi   Dar es Salaam   Cape Town
Melbourne   Auckland
and associated companies in
Berlin   Ibadan

Oxford is a trade mark of Oxford University Press

Published in the United States
by Oxford University Press, New York

© David Armstrong, Michael Calnan, and John Grace, 1990

British Library Cataloguing in Publication Data
Armstrong, David, 1947–
Research methods for general practitioners.
1. Medicine. Research. Methodology
I. Title   II. Calnan, Michael, 1949–   III. Grace,
John
610'.72
ISBN 0–19–261822–9

Library of Congress Cataloging-in-Publication Data
Armstrong, David, 1947–
Research methods for general practitioners.
(Oxford general practice series ; 16)
Includes bibliographies.
1. Medicine—Research—Methodology.   2. Physicians
(General practice)   I. Calnan, Michael.   II. Grace, John,
MRCGP.   III. Title.   IV. Series: Oxford general practice
series ; no. 16. [DNLM: 1. Family Practice.   2. Research
Design.   W1 OX55 no. 16 / W 89 A735r]
R850.A76 1989   610'.72   89–16104
ISBN 0–19–261822–9

Set by Footnote Graphics, Warminster, Wilts
Printed in Great Britain by
Biddles Ltd, Guildford & King's Lynn

Foreword

by Professor P. M. Higgins OBE MB BS FRCP FRCGP
Regional Adviser In General Practice, South East Thames Region

Like medicine—or painting—research is best learnt by doing it. Before the doing, however, comes the beginning and that is where most people stop. The value of this book is that the reader is eased into beginning without undue pain.

The book began its life as one of the region's experimental courses—one of several ventures to help general practioners (who face some of the most intractable research problems in medicine) to ask and follow up useful questions about their work and its problems. It is a collaborative effort between a general practitioner–course organizer and social scientists from two of the region's three universities.

The book is a practical, down-to-earth guide which involves the reader in performing actions that will make him or her a research worker. Its easy style engages interest; it is equally suitable for individuals or for groups and I particularly commend it to trainers who wish to help trainees acquire research skills.

Preface

Our aim in writing this book is to provide sufficient practical guidance to get you to the point where you will be able to complete and publish a research project of your own. We have therefore tried to emphasize involvement in actually doing research: in part this is through examples, but is also by various assignments:

● At various points in the text you will find *Questions*: allow yourself some time to pause at these to see if you can answer them. The text then goes on to provide answers which you can compare with your own.

● At other points you will find *Exercises*: these are meant to be a more formal assessment of what you have learned. In the first read-through you may wish to skip them but we do suggest that at some time you try and complete them. With the pressure of work you may be tempted not to complete them all, but we would urge you to try and do so because this is the best guide you will have that you have mastered that point. In addition some of the exercises will give you 'hands-on' experience of carrying out parts of the research process.

● We have also included some suggested *Tasks* at the end of every chapter, which you can carry out on your own, or more preferably with others. In fact as research is so often a group activity you might consider working through this book with others, perhaps carrying out a 'group research project' as you do so, that way you would be able to share the discussion and the work. Perhaps a trainers' workshop, young principals' group, or a trainer and trainee might find working together on a research question of mutual interest a useful way of both learning about and doing research.

THE RESEARCH PROCESS

The different stages of carrying out a research project will be covered in the various chapters of this book. In outline these stages are:

(1) Asking a question.

(2) Establishing a plan or design of how the answering is to proceed; this is the guide for all future activity.

(3) Deciding on how the various ideas expressed in the question are to be measured.

(4) The actual measuring – usually referred to as 'data collection'.

(5) Organizing the collected data into a form suitable for analysis.

(6)   Analysing the data, usually with the involvement of statistical tests.

(7)   Writing up the results.

(8)   If appropriate, finding a journal in which to publish the study.

The last chapter, on writing a research protocol, could equally well have been the first chapter because the protocol comes near the start of all research projects. In the end we thought that knowing how to begin should probably come after seeing where you were going to go: writing a protocol is therefore the final chapter of this book, but we hope that it is the beginning of your research in the rich and varied field of general practice.

London   D.A.
July 1989   M.C.
                                                                                         J.G.

Contents

1 Asking questions

This first chapter is about the most fundamental part of 'doing' research, namely, asking questions. Research attempts to answer questions: this is both very simple and very important. Possibly one of the most common reasons for research 'failing' is that there was not a proper question to start with. People often decide to 'look at' an area or problem, or they collect data about something that interests them: by and large this is wasted time. *Research must start with a question.* We cannot reiterate this point sufficiently; do not start 'doing' research until you have a question.

The difficulty with this part of the research process is that we cannot 'teach' you to ask questions—this is personal and must come from you. We can, however, provide you with some suggestions of how to start and basic guidelines to enable you to decide whether the question you ask is a good one or not, particularly whether it is answerable.

THINKING OF QUESTIONS

Research questions are often described as theories or hypotheses because they are expressed in abstract terms, as sets of ideas or concepts. These ideas are then tested in the 'real' world of facts and data. Hence science has been characterized as the 'hypothetico-deductive method' because an event is deduced from an abstract hypothesis, and the real world is then examined to see if it is there or has occurred: if it has, the hypothesis is said to have been confirmed. The hypothesis or question is thus the starting point for research and, as has been stressed, it is therefore very important. Nevertheless it is only the *formal* starting point.

In popular imagery, the scientist always starts from a question or theory which comes as a flash of inspiration, usually while in the bath or on a tram (when they were around). The reality is far less romantic. Most research questions actually arise from rather routine observed events. Doll and Hill did not suddenly think, 'Does smoking cause lung cancer?'; rather, clinicians had observed an apparent link between the behaviour and the disease in the patients they treated. This was induction: observations leading to a question. Thereafter the question was treated by the canons of scientific procedure—the hypothetico-deductive method—in that a study was set up to compare the smoking habits of patients with and without lung cancer. In fact, science moves in a continuous process of induction from experience followed by formal deduction and testing, followed by further induction, and so on.

The philosophical issues of induction and deduction lie beyond the remit of this book. The practical message is that, by and large, research questions do not come from some nebulous faculty you either do or do not possess, such as creativity or inspiration, but from everyday observations. In formulating questions, anything goes: use your clinical experience, chance findings, casual discussions, car rides, even a toy boat in the bath, but get the questions flowing. Keep a book, a diary, a list: sort them, reject some, develop others, and when you have one which you find interesting, consider putting it to the test.

Of course, having selected an interesting question one is still faced with the problem of whether the ability to answer that question is within the resources of time, money, support, etc. available to you. A 'good' research question may not be synonymous with 'a good research question for a GP' or even 'a good research question for me'.

Another important point to make is that the questions need not necessarily be complicated or difficult. It is often the simple questions that are easily overlooked, or the answers assumed:

● Are coronaries best managed in hospital?
● Is shingles contagious?
● Does physiotherapy help in the management of acute low back pain?

You don't have to be a creative genius to think of research questions. Suffice it to say that, in the largely unchartered field of primary care, a large enough number of questions or areas of doubt probably arise during the course of every working day to make the preparation of a list of questions relatively easy. That is not to say that what may appear to be easy questions to ask are necessarily easy questions to answer, but they may be. We can help you to sift your ideas so as to eliminate obviously doubtful ones. We can possibly help you work out what to do next. But it is your ability to recognize areas of doubt and turn them into good questions that will ultimately determine whether you do 'good' research, no matter how many 'techniques' you master from this book. The questions are there: just open your mind and let the questions creep in!

Exercise 1(1)

You may find it worthwhile to take a notebook with you on your next full working day. During the course of the day, jot down in the book ten questions or areas of doubt that occur to you. At the end of the day subject these questions to a critical analysis to separate out those questions which might be suitable for researching further. Evaluate them in terms of answerability and general usefulness. You could use a scale of 1 to 5 for each characteristic, marking the least answerable and the least useful as 1, and the most answerable and the most useful as 5.

Questions	Answerability	Usefulness

Question 1(1)

Which of the following questions, the sort that might occur to you during the course of a day's work, might be suitable as the basis for a research project?

(a)   Does smoking cause cancer?
(b)   Did Mr Smith take his tablets today?
(c)   Is this pain angina?
(d)   I wonder if God helps recovery from surgery?
(e)   Are antibiotics effective against viruses?
(f)   Does bed rest help in the treatment of bad backs?
(g)   Do chronic bronchitics cough up sputum?

(a)   *Does smoking cause cancer?* It is already well established and proven beyond all reasonable doubt that there is a strong association between smoking and several types of cancer. A compromise has to be reached between attempts to reinvent the wheel and a proper questioning of established but unproven practices. In this particular instance the balance would appear to be clearly on the side of the wheelsmith.

(b)   *Did Mr Smith take his tablets today?* Some questions, although possibly of interest in a particular instance, are of limited general applicability and can be considered too trivial for the use of the research method as a way of answering them.

(c)   *Is this pain angina?* This is the type of question which occurs in everyday clinical practice. However, it requires the application of the clinical, rather than the research, method. Although we shall see later that there are strong similarities in approach between the two methods, the research method is best reserved for questions which appear to have a wider application.

(d)   *I wonder if God helps recovery from surgery?* This is obviously an important question. It is also of wide application. Unfortunately, it is unanswerable as it stands under present circumstances. If it were rephrased as, 'Does a belief in God aid recovery from surgery?' then the question is limited to one of more manageable proportions, although it would then be a matter of judgement as to whether the amended question is now so altered as to have little in common with the original proposal. To reiterate, at the end of the day a good research question has to be answerable.

(e)   *Are antibiotics effective against viruses?* This really is a similar problem to that in (a). The answer is already known beyond reasonable doubt. However, your observations may lead you to question the assumed answer and formulate new hypotheses—but are you sure there is not an alternative simple explanation?

(f)   *Does bed rest help in the treatment of bad backs?* This is a question of wide general application which tests an accepted clinical practice for which there does not appear to be a lot of evidence. This could well form the basis for a useful research question.

(g)   *Do chronic bronchitics cough up sputum?* This is essentially a definitional question. The accepted definition of chronic bronchitis is based on the regular expectoration of a defined amount of sputum. Therefore there is no real question to answer.

In summary, questions can be rendered inappropriate for research because:

- The answer is already known.
- The question is not of general interest, possibly only related to one case.
- Some questions, although important, are unanswerable by research methods used and accepted at present.
- Some questions are definitional.

Let us now examine this last point in more detail.

EMPIRICAL QUESTIONS

Questions and answers can be divided into two types: *definitional*, which simply restate in other words the initial idea; and *empirical*, which potentially tell us something about the world in which we live. Karl Popper, the doyen of scientific philosophers, used this idea in his criterion of what was to count as a scientific statement or question. He decided that science consists of questions, hypotheses, and statements which are, *in principle*, refutable; that is, they have the potential to be disproved.

Be careful therefore to distinguish between these two claims to the truth. In this book we are concerned with empirical questions only, and not those that are definitional (though sometimes the latter can masquerade as the former). For example, could you investigate the claim that 'asthma causes recurrent small airways obstruction', or that 'asthma stunts growth'? Probably not the former, since if asthma did not cause recurrent small airways obstruction then it would not, by definition, be asthma; but the second hypothesis can be investigated because it could be incorrect *without* under-mining the accepted definition of asthma.

Sometimes it is unclear whether a question is 'true by definition' or empirically testable. Consider the following questions:

1. Do patients with over 95 mm Hg diastolic blood pressure have hyper-tension?
2. Are patients who appear reluctant to return to work malingerers?
3. Are diabetics with a fasting blood sugar of 8 mmol/litre adequately controlled?

In each case the question might be a definitional one, that is if hyperten-sion, malingering, and diabetic control are predefined. On the other hand, if these three phenomena are defined in some other independent way it may be possible to 'test' the question. For example, if hypertension were defined as raised blood pressure such as to increase the risk of a stroke, then it would be possible to test whether 95 mm Hg diastolic pressure was an indicator of hypertension.

Exercise 1(2)

Which of the following questions would be suitable for a research project?

(a) Do diabetics have high fasting blood sugars?
(b) Do NSAIs (non-steroidal anti-inflammatory agents) cause cancer?
(c) Are patients who complain of dizziness likely to suffer from a serious disease
(d) Are my receptionists kind to my patients?
(e) Am I working harder than my partners?
(f) Is asthma more common in only children?

Suggested answers are at the end of the chapter.

CLASSIFYING QUESTIONS

Research is often divided into three types: 'research', 'audit', and 'moni-toring'.

A distinction is often made between these three terms, the implication being that they form a hierarchy of enquiry.

Monitoring is seen as a form of counting. It allows one to describe what is happening, but no more.

Audit is usually taken to mean a measurement of performance against a predetermined set of standards. For example, one could decide that for a diagnosis of hypertension to be confirmed, three readings of a diastolic pressure over 100 mm Hg on three separate occasions were required. An auditing exercise of all the patients on anti-hypertensive treatment could be carried out, in order to determine to what extent this preset standard for the diagnosis had been satisfied.

Research is an activity with certain rules, which involves questioning, setting hypotheses, and then devising methods that seek to support or refute these hypotheses.

Confusion between the terms audit and research is often found. Research is occasionally taken to imply purely a difference in scope of enquiry, rather than type of enquiry when compared with audit. An editorial in the *Journal of the Royal College of General Practitioners* suggested that 'Research provides information which has relevance and value beyond the particular circumstances of the study. In contrast, audit aims to provide precise information in a particular setting which enables rational policy decisions to be made.' It is clear that here the author is more concerned with size and applicability than with any inherent differences in definitions.

So although there is some confusion, and possible misuse of the three terms, especially of the word 'research', we would hope that one of the aims of this book will be to encourage you to try all three forms of enquiry within your own capabilities. Hopefully the relationship between the three will become clearer as you progress through the book.

Exercise 1(3)

Using the above classification, into what types of research would you put the folowing questions?

(a)   What is the age-sex structure of the practice?
(b)   How many prescriptions did I issue in the past month?
(c)   Does recent unemployment make patients attend more often?
(d)   Is my appointment system operating satisfactorily?
(e)   Do people who have to look after dependent relations at home consult more often?
(f)   Are the immunization rates for my 5-year-olds satisfying the district norms?

Suggested answers are at the end of the chapter.

EXPLORING THE QUESTION

Having identified a possibly 'good' research question, the next stage is to investigate the background of the question before we can move on to researching an answer with some confidence. Has someone else had a go at answering it? Is the answer known? Has someone formulated it in a better way?

In addition, this exploratory phase will be useful for the very final stages of the research process, namely in writing up for publication, in that a journal article usually opens with some discussion of the background to the question, together with an overview of existing literature (see Chapter 9).

Let us examine the background to a simple question:

Question 1(2)

Are antibiotics of value in the treament of acute otitis media?

(a)   Yes.
(b)   No.
(c)   Sometimes.

Consider the grounds you have for holding your opinion, the degree of certainty with which you hold it, and possible sources of knowledge. How could you find out whether an adequate answer already exists for this or any other particular problem? There are many fairly readily available sources of knowledge which we all use from time to time, depending on the question being asked and the degree of faith we have in the received answer.

1.   Ask a GP or colleague? This is easy, and possibly the most widely used method; but how reliable is it? Is the opinion of a colleague likely to be based on similar false assumptions to your own?

2.   Look it up in a textbook? Textbooks are extremely useful and again fairly readily available sources of information. They vary greatly in standard and size, depending partly on the audience for which they were designed. A 100-page 'Concise Illustrated Textbook of Ear, Nose and Throat Medicine for students and GPs' has to sacrifice for the sake of brevity certain aspects of erudition that a 1000-page 'Textbook on Disease of the Human Cochlea' does not. Shorter tomes are more likely to be a synopsis of common practice rather than validated current knowledge. They are rarely referenced, which makes it difficult, if not impossible, for the reader to check the information presented. All textbooks suffer from preparation-lag; the often considerable delay between the writing and the publishing means that the information can be anything up to two years out of date on the day the brand-new textbook is published.

3.   Ask a consultant colleague in the field? This is likely to produce a more authoritative opinion or answer than asking a non-specialist colleague. A specialist's opinion should also be based on more recent developments or information than textbooks—on the assumption that specialists read specialists' journals. But can you be any more certain that it is more reliable? If his opinion is backed by references that can be checked, then one might perhaps be less suspicious but, unfortunately, people develop ways of behaving and doing things which they find comfortable. Doctors are no exception. Many become entrapped in a mode of unques-

tioning behaviour where doubt does not assume a prominent place. Comments about the level of research activity in primary care, and among general practitioners in particular, could probably as readily be made about in-post consultants outside academic units. Indeed, very few aspects of clinical practice have ever been subjected to proper scientific evaluation. With these reservations in mind it may be that specialists are a source of information that needs to be subjected to as much critical assessment as any other.

4.   Carry out a literature review? To find the current state of play about most medical problems one is forced to 'search the literature'—that is, either to find a detailed critical review article on a subject with references appended, or to look up the original article itself and to make some evaluative assessment of that article, especially in relation to the specific problem you have in mind. This usually entails spending time in your local postgraduate centre library. These, of course, vary greatly in size and shape. A possible minimal criterion of the adequacy of your local postgraduate centre library would be whether or not it has a qualified librarian. If it has not, then we suggest you find the nearest one that has. Librarians are highly trained specialists in finding things out, and a few minutes discussing the problem you are trying to solve with a libarian may well increase the efficiency of the time you actually spend searching in the library many times over. Get to know your library and the facilities it offers, it is a valuable resource.

The librarian will probably introduce you to two main methods of searching through the literature.

Manual searches

This is normally done by looking up the topic in *Cumulated Index Medicus*. This is an index, or list, of all papers published in the major medical journals throughout the world. It appears monthly, with yearly compilations, catalogued by both subject and author. The use of *Index Medicus* involves:

● Finding the right synonym for the keyword or words, under which heading papers relating to your particular query might be filed.
● Looking at this keyword in the subject headings. It is especially worth looking for review articles in the leading and readily available journals (e.g. *British Medical Journal, Journal of the Royal College of General Practitioners, Lancet*, etc.). Once into these articles a form of journal daisy-chaining can be started. The particular article is looked up in the named journal, and then further papers listed in the references list at the end of the article can be examined. One or two might be obtained

and the reference lists of these in turn can be looked at, the papers examined and so on, and so on.

Obviously papers in the English language, and especially British journals will be easier to obtain, but the librarian should be able to obtain a copy of most papers on request.

For example, to answer the question of whether antibiotics are of value in the treatment of otitis media we might follow the following procedure.

Look up the keyword 'otitis media'. This was done using the *Cumulated Index Medicus* for 1985. In a sub-division of the entries under 'otitis media', subtitled 'drug therapy', were found six articles that seemed to address the question posed. Two of these, an original article and a letter criticizing the article, were in the *British Medical Journal*, which is commonly available in most medical libraries. The references at the bottom of this article produced further articles, and further reference lists, and so on.

Figures 1.1 and 1.2 illustrate this procedure.

Computerized literature searches

This is the age of the technological and information revolution. As well as blasting aliens, the computer in its spare time has been used for the storage of vast amounts of information and, more importantly, allowed ready access to and searching of this information. This facility has been seized upon by those engaged in compiling catalogues such as the *Index Medicus*.

There are several of these computerized data-bases solely restricted to medical literature. Many postgraduate centre libraries have facilities to plug into one of these centralized lists by using a computer terminal in the library and a telephone line connecting it to a large computer, often many thousands of miles away. The Royal College of General Practitioners provides a similar facility to both members and non-members (at different rates) with their ON-LINE SEARCH SERVICE. All these services provide a rapid search of a wide range of literature. They do have problems however:

- They cost money to use.
- The efficient use of the facility requires the correct selection of keywords. These are similar to those required for the manual use of the *Index Medicus*, but need, if anything, to be even more specific and exact. For example using the keywords 'ENT' and 'General Practice' to search the literature in the otitis media problem would provide a list of references of every publication on file, for as far back as has been computerized, in which any aspect of ENT was connected with any aspect of general practice.

The selection of the correct keywords is therefore the secret to using

1985 **CUMULATED INDEX MEDICUS** **OTITIS MEDIA**

PG. **Mykosen** 1985 May;28(5):234–7

Bacteriologic studies in external otitis in Dar es Salaam, Tanzania. Manni JJ, et al. **Trop Geogr Med** 1984 Sep; 36(3):293–5

PARASITOLOGY

[Human otoacariasis caused by Otobius megnini in Calama, Chile] Burchard L, et al. **Bol Chil Parasitol** 1984 Jan-Jun; 39(1-2):15-6 (Eng. Abstr.) **(Spa)**

PATHOLOGY

Bilateral chondrodermatitis helicis: case presentation and literature review. Cannon CR. **Am J Otol** 1985 Mar; 6(2):164–6

RADIOGRAPHY

Radiologic abnormalities of malignant otitis externa. Pripstein S, et al. **Rev Laryngol Otol Rhinol (Bord)** 1984; 105(3):307-10

Radiologic evaluation of malignant external otitis. Smoker WR, et al. **Rev Laryngol Otol Rhinol (Bord)** 1984; 105(3):297-301

RADIONUCLIDE IMAGING

The radionuclide diagnosis, evaluation and follow-up of malignant external otitis (MEO). The value of immediate blood pool scanning. Garty I, et al. **J Laryngol Otol** 1985 Feb;99(2):109-15

RADIOTHERAPY

[Low-energy laser irradiation in the complex treatment of patients with ear diseases] Bykov VL, et al. **Vopr Kurortol Fizioter Lech Fiz Kult** 1985 Mar-Apr; (2):60–2 **(Rus)**

THERAPY

Prognostic implications of therapy for necrotizing external otitis [clinical conference] Corey JP, et al. **Am J Otol** 1985 Jul;6(4):353-8

Surgical applications of the expandable ear wick. Cannon CR. **Laryngoscope** 1985 Jun;95(6):739–40

VETERINARY

Mycotic otitis externa in animals. Kuttin ES, et al. **Mykosen** 1985 Feb;28(2):61-8

OTITIS MEDIA

Experimental otitis media with effusion. Proceedings of the international conference, Lövångers Kyrkstad, August 17-20, 1983. **Acta Otolaryngol [Suppl] (Stockh)** 1984; 414:1-188

Recent advances in otitis media with effusion. Report of research conference. Fort Lauderdale, May 20-21, 1983. **Ann Otol Rhinol Laryngol [Suppl]** 1985 Jan-Feb;116:1-32

A 5-year prospective case-control study of the influence of early otitis media with effusion on reading achievement. Lous J, et al. **Int J Pediatr Otorhinolaryngol** 1984 Oct; 8(1):19-30

Persistent and recurrent otitis media. A review of the 'otitis-prone' condition. Berman S, et al. **Primary Care** 1984 Sep;11(3):407-17 (57 ref.)

[Serous-mucoid otitis media in infants] Narcy P, et al. **Ann Pediatr (Paris)** 1984 Dec;31(11):939–43 (Eng. Abstr.) **(Fre)**

[Otitis media in the newborn infant: cytologic and bacteriologic study and long-term results] Pestalozza G, et al. **Acta Otorhinolaryngol Ital** 1984 Jan-Feb;4(1):27–47 (Eng. Abstr.) **(Ita)**

BLOOD

Subclinical trace element deficiency in children with undue susceptibility to infections. Bondestam M, et al. **Acta Paediatr Scand** 1985 Jul;74(4):515-20

Similar hematologic changes in children receiving trimethoprim-sulfamethoxazole or amoxicillin for otitis media. Feldman S, et al. **J Pediatr** 1985 Jun;106(6):995-1000

CHEMICALLY INDUCED

[Carrageenins-induced otitis media in animal] Shibahara Y, et al. **Nippon Jibiinkoka Gakkai Kaiho** 1984 Jun;87(6):680–7 (Eng. Abstr.) **(Jpn)**

COMPLICATIONS

Middle ear disease in samples from the general population. II. History of otitis and otorrhea in relation to tympanic membrane pathology. The study of men born in 1913 and 1923. Rudin R, et al. **Acta Otolaryngol (Stockh)** 1985 Jan-Feb;99(1-2):53-9

Intracranial complications of otitis media. Debruyne F. **Acta Otorhinolaryngol Belg** 1984;38(2):128-32

Characteristics of earache among children with acute otitis media. Hayden GF, et al. **Am J Dis Child** 1985 Jul; 139(7):721-3

The frequency of vestibular disorders in developmentally delayed preschoolers with otitis media. Schaaf RC. **Am J Occup Ther** 1985 Apr;39(4):247-52

Subarachnoid space: middle ear pathways and recurrent meningitis. Barcz DV, et al. **Am J Otol** 1985 Mar; 6(2):157–63

The etiologic role of acute suppurative otitis media in chronic secretory otitis. Stangerup SE, et al. **Am J Otol** 1985 Mar; 6(2):126-31

Sensorineural hearing loss in otitis media. Paparella MM, et al. **Ann Otol Rhinol Laryngol** 1984 Nov-Dec;93(6 Pt 1):623-9

Ventilating tubes in the middle ear. Long-term observations. Gundersen T, et al. **Arch Otolaryngol** 1984 Dec; 110(12):783–4

Analysis of fifty cases of facial palsy due to otitis media. Takahashi H, et al. **Arch Otorhinolaryngol** 1985; 241(2):163-8

Otitis media: the role of speech-language pathologists. Garrard KR, et al. **ASHA** 1985 Jul;27(7):35-9

The minimally hearing-impaired child. Bess FH. **Ear Hear** 1985 Jan-Feb;6(1):43-7

Basal cell carcinoma following chronic otitis media. Myskowski PL, et al. **Int J Dermatol** 1985 Mar;24(2):120–1

Brain abscess secondary to otitis media. Bradley PJ, et al. **J Laryngol Otol** 1984 Dec;98(12):1185-91

Lateral sinus thrombosis in the eighties. Debruyne F. **J Laryngol Otol** 1985 Jan;99(1):91-3

Otologic features of bacterial meningitis of childhood. Eavey RD, et al. **J Pediatr** 1985 Mar;106(3):402-7

Relationship between acute suppurative otitis media and chronic secretory otitis media: role of antibiotics. Mills R, et al. **J R Soc Med** 1984 Sep;77(9):754-7

Otitic hydrocephalus. Lenz RP, et al. **Laryngoscope** 1984 Nov;94(11 Pt 1):1451–4

Acute mastoiditis complicated by bacterial meningitis. Braverman AC, et al. **Mo Med** 1985 Jun;82(6):308-11

Purulent otitis media--a 'silent' source of sepsis in the pediatric intensive care unit. Persico M, et al. **Otolaryngol Head Neck Surg** 1985 Jun;93(3):330–4

Postinflammatory ossicular fixation: CT analysis with surgical correlation. Swartz JD, et al. **Radiology** 1985 Mar; 154(3):697-700

Intracranial complications of ear disease in a pediatric population with special emphasis on subdural effusion and empyema. Gower DJ, et al. **South Med J** 1985 Apr; 78(4):429-34

[Results of tympanometry in infantile allergic rhinopathy] Corrias A, et al. **Minerva Pediatr** 1984 Nov 30; 36(22):1115-8 (Eng. Abstr.) **(Ita)**

[Otogenic intracranial complications--an ever-present problem] Janczewski G, et al. **Otolaryngol Pol** 1985; 39(1):7-18 (Eng. Abstr.) **(Pol)**

[Chronic purulent otitis media complicated by an extensive phlegmon of the neck] Bystrenin AV. **Vestn Otorinolaringol** 1985 May-Jun;(3):79-80 **(Rus)**

[Roentgenological diagnosis of labyrinthine fistulas in chronic suppurative otitis media] Kossovoi AL. **Vestn Otorinolaringol** 1985 Jan-Feb;(1):17-20 (Eng. Abstr.) **(Rus)**

[Social rehabilitation of patients in the late period after surgery for an otogenic brain abscess] Markin SA, et al. **Vestn Otorinolaringol** 1985 May-Jun;(3):36-9 (Eng. Abstr.) **(Rus)**

[Otogenic brain abscess in a child] Sal'nikova EA, et al. **Vestn Otorinolaringol** 1985 Mar-Apr;(2):58-60 **(Rus)**

[Cerebrovascular disorders and ischemic stroke in patients with chronic suppurative otitis media, simulating otogenic intracranial complications] Shuster MA, et al. **Vestn Otorinolaringol** 1985 Jan-Feb;(1):41-4 (Eng. Abstr.) **(Rus)**

DIAGNOSIS

Otitis media in early infancy. Papadeas VA, et al. **Am J Emerg Med** 1984 May;2(3):251-3

Aboriginal child health. Stuart J. **Aust Fam Physician** 1985 Jul;14(7):677-80

Follow-up visit after acute otitis media. Puczynski MS, et al. **Br J Clin Pract** 1985 Apr;39(4):132-4, 153

Ear wax and otitis media in children. Fairey A, et al. **Br Med J [Clin Res]** 1985 Aug 10;291(6492):387-8

Study of middle ear disease using tympanometry in general practice. Reves R, et al. **Br Med J [Clin Res]** 1985 Jun 29;290(6486):1953-6

Age-specific patterns of diagnosis of acute otitis media. McFadden DM, et al. **Clin Pediatr (Phila)** 1985 Oct; 24(10):571-5

Otitis media in newborn infants. Pestalozza G. **Int J Pediatr Otorhinolaryngol** 1984 Dec;8(2):109-24

Acoustic impedance measurement as screening procedure in children: discussion paper. Brooks DN. **J R Soc Med** 1985 Feb;78(2):119-21

Screening for middle ear fluid in an urban pre-school population. Paulman PM, et al. **Nebr Med J** 1984 Sep; 69(9):307

Acoustic reflectometry in the detection of middle ear effusion. Lampe RM, et al. **Pediatrics** 1985 Jul;76(1):75-8

[Acute inflammation of the middle ear] Feenstra L. **Ned Tijdschr Geneeskd** 1985 Mar 23;129(12):532-6 **(Dut)**

[Tympanometry under nitrous oxide anesthesia in cases of seromucous otitis] Coeckelenbergh A, et al. **Acta Otorhinolaryngol Belg** 1984;38(5):485-8 (Eng. Abstr.) **(Fre)**

[Embryonal rhabdomyosarcoma of the middle ear and mastoid simulating chronic otitis media] Shohet I, et al. **Harefuah** 1984 Nov 15;107(10):290–1 (Eng. Abstr.) **(Heb)**

[A case of aspergillosis of the ear] Sekula J, et al. **Otolaryngol Pol** 1985;39(2):166–70 (Eng. Abstr.) **(Pol)**

[Differential diagnostic problems in diseases and injuries of the middle ear] Kitanoski B, et al. **Vojnosanit Pregl** 1985 Jan-Feb;42(1):14–8 (Eng. Abstr.) **(Scr)**

DRUG THERAPY

Efficacy of Metronidazole in experimental Bacteroides fragilis otitis media. Thore M, et al. **Acta Otolaryngol (Stockh)** 1985 Jan-Feb;99(1-2):60–6

Acute otitis media in older children and adults treated with penicillin or erythromycin. Rosén C, et al. **Acta Otolaryngol [Suppl] (Stockh)** 1984;407:23-5

Antibiotic treatment of secretory otitis media. Sundberg L. **Acta Otolaryngol [Suppl] (Stockh)** 1984;407:26–9

Improving compliance with antibiotic regimens for otitis media. Randomized clinical trial in a pediatric clinic. Finney JW, et al. **Am J Dis Child** 1985 Jan;139(1):89–95

Erythromycin-sulfisoxazole vs amoxicillin in the treatment of acute otitis media in children. A double-blind, multiple-dose comparative study. Rodriguez WJ, et al. **Am J Dis Child** 1985 Aug;139(8):766–70

Drugs affecting clearance of middle ear secretions: a perspective for the management of otitis media with effusion. Brown DT, et al. **Ann Otol Rhinol Laryngol [Suppl]** 1985 Mar-Apr;117:3-15

Acute otitis media: a new treatment strategy [letter] **Br Med J [Clin Res]** 1985 Jun 8;290(6483):1743–4

Acute otitis media: a new treatment strategy. van Buchem FL, et al. **Br Med J [Clin Res]** 1985 Apr 6;290(6474):1033-7

The 'new' ampicillins: who needs them? Committee on Infectious Diseases and Immunization, Canadian Paediatric Society. **Can Med Assoc J** 1984 Nov 15;131(10):1223–4

Bromhexine in the treatment of otitis media with effusion. Stewart IA, et al. **Clin Otolaryngol** 1985 Jun;10(3):145-9

The long-term outcome of nonsuppurative otitis media with effusion. Dusdieker LB, et al. **Clin Pediatr (Phila)** 1985 Apr; 24(4):181-6

Fungal infection of the ear. Etiology and therapy with bifonazole cream or solution. Falser N. **Dermatologica** 1984; 169 Suppl 1:135–40

Oral nystatin [letter] Crook WG. **Ear Nose Throat J** 1985 Mar;64(3):155

Otitis media: treatment and side effects [letter] Crook WG. **Hosp Pract [Off]** 1985 Sep 30;20(9A):14, 16

Antimicrobial therapy of chronic otitis media with effusion. Healy GB. **Int J Pediatr Otorhinolaryngol** 1984 Oct; 8(1):13-7

Compliance with acute otitis media treatment. Reed BD, et al. **J Fam Pract** 1984 Nov;19(5):627-32

A randomized controlled trial of cefaclor compared with trimethoprim-sulfamethoxazole for treatment of acute otitis media. Marchant CD, et al. **J Pediatr** 1984 Oct;105(4):633-8

Mucolytic agents for glue ear [letter] Pearson JP, et al. **Lancet** 1985 Sep 21;2(8456):674

Trimet v amoxycillin in the treatment of otitis media in children [letter] Godfrey AA, et al. **NZ Med J** 1985 Apr 10;98(776):252

Medical management of serous otitis media. Crysdale WS. **Otolaryngol Clin North Am** 1984 Nov;17(4):653-7

Medical management of chronic otitis media. Jahn AF, et al. **Otolaryngol Clin North Am** 1984 Nov;17(4):673-7

Occurrence of Clostridium difficile toxin-associated gastroenteritis following antibiotic therapy for otitis media in young children. Hyams JS, et al. **Pediatr Infect Dis** 1984 Sep–Oct;3(5):433-6

In vivo sensitivity test in otitis media: efficacy of antibiotics. Howie VM, et al. **Pediatrics** 1985 Jan;75(1):8-13

Oral dexamethasone for treatment of persistent middle ear effusion. Macknin ML, et al. **Pediatrics** 1985 Feb; 75(2):329-35

Comparative treatment trial of augmentin versus cefaclor for acute otitis media with effusion. Odio CM, et al. **Pediatrics** 1985 May;75(5):819-26

Trimethoprim and amoxycillin in acute otitis media. Backhouse CI, et al. **Practitioner** 1985 Jan;229(1399):51–4

[Adapting the therapy to the course of acute otitis media] van Buchem FL, et al. **Ned Tijdschr Geneeskd** 1985 Jun 8;129(23):1093-9 (Eng. Abstr.) **(Dut)**

[Effect of Tavegyl (Polfa) on microorganisms detected in otocenosis during in vivo studies] Kurnatowski P, et al. **Otolaryngol Pol** 1984;38(3):219-24 (Eng. Abstr.) **(Pol)**

[Use of lekozim in middle ear diseases] Tarasov DI, et al. **Vestn Otorinolaringol** 1985 May-Jun;(3):43-7 (Eng. Abstr.) **(Rus)**

ENZYMOLOGY

Biochemical pathology of otitis media with effusion. Juhn SK, et al. **Acta Otolaryngol [Suppl] (Stockh)** 1984;414:45-51

Hydrolase activity in acute otitis media with effusion. Diven WF, et al. **Ann Otol Rhinol Laryngol** 1985 Jul-Aug;94(4 Pt 1):415-8

Antifibrinolytic activity in middle ear effusion. Hamaguchi Y, et al. **ORL J Otorhinolaryngol Relat Spec** 1984; 46(5):235–41

[Lysosomal enzyme activity in middle ear effusions] Hara A, et al. **Nippon Jibiinkoka Gakkai Kaiho** 1984 May; 87(5):596–602 (Eng. Abstr.) **(Jpn)**

ETIOLOGY

Endotoxin in middle ear effusions tested with Limulus assay.

12621

Fig. 1.1 Finding the references.

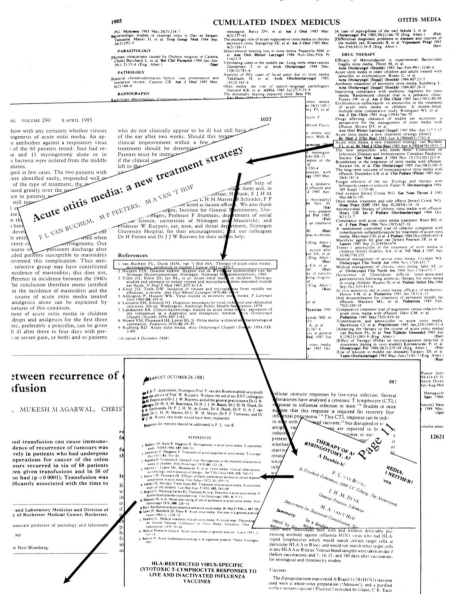

Fig. 1.2. Reference daisy-chaining.

these data-bases. Again, the librarian can be of enormous value in the proper selection of these keywords and the saving of your time and expense.

The medical librarian at a post-graduate centre was asked to produce a list of references which might help answer the question posed. The search was carried out on Medline, one of several computerized data-bases, using the keywords *otitis media* and *antibiotics*. The search was restricted to English-language journals for the past 5 years. It produced 52 articles.

Question 1(3)

What might be the respective advantages and disadvantages of manual and computerized literature searches?

The manual method might be expected to be time-consuming and prone to errors. However, it allows discrimination in ignoring articles which address questions other than those in which one is directly interested: e.g. Is drug A better than drug B in otitis media? Is 10 days of drug C better than 3 days?

It also allows one to ignore journals which are not immediately accessible. In the exercise described above, it was possible to identify two papers within 10 minutes, by van Buchem in the *BMJ* and the *Lancet*, that appeared directly to address the question posed. The computerized search might be expected to be quicker and more thorough. In fact it took over a week to get the list back on account of the pressure of work on the librarian, would have cost between £10 and £20 at current prices, produced a far more comprehensive list, but in the end probably only nine of the 52 papers were specifically looking at the question in hand; and for some reason it missed one important paper (the van Buchem paper in the *BMJ*) which the manual search turned up. You pays your money and takes your choice.

As always, a compromise is available. At some 'well-resourced', not to say well-heeled medical libraries, the *Index Medicus* has recently become available on compact discs—in between Dire Straits and Shostakovitch! When these are used along with suitable equipment and a personal computer, it allows for a far quicker search—more limited in scope than the traditional computer search, but probably potentially better than a manual search.

Exercise 1(4)

If you have not already done so, take the opportunity in the near future of visiting your local postgraduate centre library and introduce yourself to the librarian. Discuss how you should set about answering the question of whether antibiotics are of value in the treatment of otitis media.

Search the literature, either manually, electronically, or both, to find which papers have been published in the last year in English-language journals on two of the following:

(a)   A subject of your own choice.
(b)   The treament of anxiety in general practice.
(c)   Screening for glaucoma.
(d)   The use of practice nurses.
(e)   Patient access to their own medical records.

Searching by whichever method you choose, should allow you to see if there already exists an answer to a question which has entered your mind. Colleagues, textbooks, specialists, and even original papers must be carefully scrutinized and critically evaluated before deciding that your particular question has been insufficiently investigated.

Question 1(4)

Take a few minutes before finishing this chapter to note down your answers to the following:

(a)   What are the benefits from *my* doing research?
(b)   What stops *me* doing research?

IT'S EASIER THAN YOU THINK

There are many reasons why people undertake research. Some feel it necessary continually to question established practices, others see it almost as a means of confirming their faith in an organized, rational world of cause and effect. Again it might be seen as a challenge, a form of intellectual nourishment. Obviously there are some who do it just for fun, or to give a wider horizon to the daily work they do. It could also be thought by some to be a form of self-discipline needed to improve personal performance – or that the nature of experiment will help develop powers of imagination and critical sense. Of course most of us do it for fame, fortune, and foreign travel! Although fortune is extremely unlikely, there is a great deal of personal satisfaction to be gained from the development of a question into a research project leading to the production of a paper and its publication in a recognized medical or scientific journal—hardly fame, but much pleasure. And while there is no guarantee of foreign travel you will at least get out to visit your local postgraduate centre. Why, then, do not more people do research?

Can it be that they are all too lazy or apathetic? Is it just that they lack research skills and knowledge of research methods? Is it that research is considered irrelevant to daily life—a thing apart to satisfy the egos of those who indulge in it?

If, indeed, a major stumbling block is the lack of research skills, or even a fundamental disbelief in the research method as a means of developing understanding, then perhaps it would be helpful to examine similarities between the research method and the clinical method taught in medical schools, and still almost universally used when doctors see patients.

Let us consider similarities between the two methods:

Research method	*Clinical method*
● Problems identified	● Problem identified (through patient's complaint)
● Formulating hypotheses	● Hypothesis formulation to explain observations (differential diagnosis)
● Testing hypotheses	● Testing (examination of patient, other investigations, effect of treatments)
● Conclusions	● Conclusions (diagnosis)
	● Follow up

There are strong similarities between the clinical method we use every day and the research method. The patient presents facts to the doctor (the presenting complaint). Almost immediately the doctor begins to arrange these facts in his or her mind, and starts to construct hypotheses to explain these facts. Testing takes place by asking more direct questions (history of the presenting condition).

> Patient: 'Doctor, I've had this pain in my chest for a couple of weeks.'
> (Hypotheses: This pain could be cardiac in origin. This pain could be muscular. This pain could be pleuritic. This pain could be anxiety, etc.).
> Doctor: 'When does it tend to occur?'
> (Testing several loose hypotheses at once.)
> Patient: 'Mainly at night when I lie down.'
> (Conclusion: less likely to be cardiac. Hypothesis: This pain could be reflux oesophagitis.)
> Doctor: 'Does it occur at any other time—with food, coughing, bending over, for example?'
> (Testing new hypothesis as well as others.)

The verbal examination will produce a set of hypotheses which are tested by the physical examination, then redefined or reconstructed and perhaps retested by the ordering of special investigations (e.g. in this example, chest X-ray, ECG, barium swallow, etc.) and possibly by the prescribing of a specific remedy (e.g. antacid). A conclusion is then reached after a period of time (which in itself is often an important test of some hypotheses in general practice), as to whether one of the hypotheses has been sufficiently supported. If the conclusion is that it has not, then the process begins again.

And despite what would appear to be a fairly marked 'similarity' between the research method and the clinical method, GPs and consultants still shy away from doing research on the grounds of professed ignorance of its method!

SUMMARY

In this chapter we have looked at the meaning of research and how it could fit into the working pattern of every thinking health-care professional. We have explored the different types of questions that can be asked and how they might be sifted. Finally, ways to check to what extent the answer is known have been described.

SUGGESTED TASKS

1.   Research can be an isolated business. Try to find out what local research facilities and support is available. Is there a local university or college with skills which you might call upon for help and advice?

2.   Is there any research actually going on locally? Try asking the following groups:

(a)   the FPC;
(b)   the District Health Authority;
(c)   the LMC; and
(d)   trainer workshops and young principals' groups.

3.   Persuade some other GPs to each bring six possible research questions to a meeting at which their feasibility and interest would be evaluated.

ANSWERS TO EXERCISES

Exercise 1(2)

(a)   No. This is a tautologous question. Diabetes is defined in terms of raised fasting blood sugars.

(b)   Yes. The answer is not immediately apparent, although it may exist within the literature. The question *is* important, the prescribing of NSAIs is common, and the question has obvious general application.

(c)   Yes. Again, the question concerns a common area of concern, has a general application, and is testable.

(d) No. The question is important, is testable, but is of little general application. However, within this constraint the balance may still lead one to want to answer the question as it stands—so the answer could be 'yes'.

(e) No. The arguments are the same as the previous question: possibly important, possibly testable, but of no general application.

(f) Yes. The question concerns a common condition, is testable, has general application, and obviously may lead onto further questions.

Exercise 1(3)

(a) Monitoring.

(b) Monitoring.

(c) Hypothesis testing (research).

(d) Audit.

(e) Hypothesis testing (research).

(f) Audit.

2 Designing a research project

Chapter 1 looked at the types of research questions that can be asked, and at ways to check to what extent the answer was known. Once you have decided on the research question(s) you need to identify the design that will be appropriate for answering them. Let us work through some examples, showing how different types of research design can be devised for different types of question.

Most GPs are committed to health education and try, when the opportunity arises, to give advice to patients during the consultation. Dr Philip Tipps is particularly interested in health education about smoking and would like to know how far the information and advice that he gives influences his patients' level of understanding, attitudes and actual smoking habits. He has therefore drawn up the following research questions:

Q. *Does the advice that I give to cigarette smokers actually change:*
- *their awareness?*
- *their attitudes?*
- *their smoking behaviour?*

Before Dr Tipps plunges into attempting to devise a study to answer these questions he visits his local postgraduate library to look up the latest edition of *The General Household Survey*, an annual report from the Office of Population Surveys and Censuses based on a national sample of households. There he discovers, amongst data on the leisure activities and health habits of the population, that about 30 per cent of the national population are current smokers, but he is not sure how far his own patients are similar to or different from the national population. Thus, he concludes that his research will require the answers to two further supplementary questions:

Q. *What proportion of my patients are current cigarette smokers?*

Q. *Who are the smokers?*

Each of these questions seems well defined, fairly specific and, above all, answerable. The next step is to devise a blueprint for how the question(s) will be answered—this is called the research design.

WHAT IS THE RESEARCH DESIGN?

The research *question* is expressed in ideas and concepts, whereas the research *design* is the plan of how the research will be carried out. It tends not to deal with specifics, but rather addresses the broad strategy of how the research will seek to answer the question. Deciding on the research design is an important procedure:

- It must enable the question to be answered; get it wrong and no matter what follows your results will not be able to answer your question.
- It must also try to rule out 'alternative answers' to the research question.

It is at this stage you might find that what you thought were 'answerable' questions are in fact unanswerable because you cannot devise a practical research design within your resource constraints. Ideally the research should create a design to fit with the research question, but in practice you might have to amend your question to fit in with the feasibility of the research design. This revision of research questions, sometimes as a result of other influences such as the knowledge gained through the literature review, is acceptable as long as you do not entirely lose sight of the original problem.

The next stage of Dr Tipps research into health education about smoking in general practice, therefore, involves him in deciding on a research design which is appropriate for each question. As we shall see, different research questions require different designs.

Q. 'What proportion of my patients are current cigarette smokers?'

The words or phrases in the research question often suggest the sort of research design required. In this instance there are four words or phases which give clues to the type of design required:

1.   By focusing on *patients* the question defines the population on which the research will be based, although there is still a decision about whether to restrict further the defined population by other criteria, such as age. For example, there are few smokers under the age of 14 but, on the other hand, the researcher may be particularly interested in this group.

2.   By focusing on whether the patient is a *smoker or not*, the research question aims to divide the patient population into two on the grounds of whether they do or do not behave in a specific way.

3.   By focusing on *what proportion* of the patient population are smokers, there is the implication that only a description of the patient population is needed, rather than an explanation of, say, why they smoke.

4.   By focusing on *current* smoking behaviour, the research question implies that information about smoking should be based on the most up-to-date sources.

In summary, the research question has told Dr Tipps that the design required should provide a descriptive profile of one characteristic of the current behaviour of a defined patient population.

Let's look at each of these aspects of the research design in turn.

Defining the population

One of the first decisions to be made is where the information about patients' smoking habits is to be found. In principle the question is answered by asking all patients whether they smoke or not. But how do you get hold of 'all patients' – they are never all collected together in one place? Various lists of all patients are available, so instead of collecting them physically together Dr Tipps could write to each individually and collect all their replies.

Question 2(1)

Dr Tipps would like to know which of his patients smoke. In order to look at this problem he realizes that he needs to know *who* his patients are. He decides that he has three sources, or sampling frames, for such a list:

(a)   the medical record envelopes;
(b)   the age–sex register his keen trainee insisted on two years ago, which has remained untouched since;
(c)   the FPC register.

What are the advantages and disadvantages of each?

   (a)   Obviously the record envelopes are unwieldly, are arranged alphabetically, and probably contain many records of patients who have either died, moved, or been transferred, or they may be lying in the back of a partner's car (the records that is, not the patients).

   (b)   Dr Tipp's own age–sex register has lain undisturbed for two years, and although it is much more convenient to handle, and is arranged chronologically, it will be grossly inaccurate by now. Even age–sex registers in well-organized practices have been found to be between 5 and 10% inaccurate when checked against FPC registers.

   (c)   The FPC, especially if computerized, may be able to provide the most up-to-date list of patients, but again will be subject to significant inflation due to the problem of belated and slow withdrawal of patients – again evidence suggests around 10% inaccuracy in FPC lists.

Exercise 2(1)

If Dr Tipps had wanted to extend his survey to include the whole population of the small town, in which his was one of four practices, where might he have been able to obtain his population list? Three common sources are:

(a)   telephone directory;
(b)   electoral register;
(c)   rating records (for households rather than individuals) or poll tax records.

What do you think might be the problems in using each? Suggested answers are at the end of the chapter.

How do you establish which patients smoke?

Having established the population, the next stage is to separate smokers from non-smokers. Had Dr Tipps been using his medical record cards as his population list, he could have checked through them to identify smoking habits—though it is doubtful if smoking behaviour would have been recorded in all, or indeed many, of them. Therefore, if the information is not already available, he will have to collect it anew.

He could send out a letter to all his patients. This would give him the 'best' result, if they all replied. However, research is not only about getting valid results it is also about being efficient in the light of the original question. The question is about a proportion who smoked, not about whether or not a particular patient smoked. There may, therefore, be easier ways of obtaining the information about a population than by asking every individual. The solution is to ask a *representative sample* of the total population if they smoke. So long as the sample is representative, i.e. has identical characteristics to that of the total population, then one can reasonably generalize from the results of that sample to the whole population: what is true for the sample should be true for the population.

The advantages of using a sample are:

(1)   it is more efficient in that it generally saves money, labour and time;

(2)   with fewer cases it is easier to collect and deal with more detailed information from each case.

On these grounds, Dr Tipps decides to select a sample. But how does he do this? The next section will examine sampling in some detail before returning to the research questions on smoking.

SAMPLING

There are various types of sample. At the end of this chapter you should know the difference between some important samples, namely *random*, *systematic*, *stratified*, and *quota*.

Question 2(2)

Dr Tipps is fortunate in that he already has an age–sex register, which, unbeknown to him, his practice manager has recently updated and corrected in line with the list held by the FPC. This is held on the Royal College of General Practitioners' age–sex cards in two tin files, one containing details of all the male patients, the other details of all the females.

He decides to use these patient lists as the source from which to draw his sample, and therefore one weekend he takes the two tins home. A quick count of the cards reveals that he has 1200 male and 1300 female patients. He further decides to take a 10% sample of the patients aged 16 and over, which works out at 85 men and 95 women.

The method he first chooses is to close his eyes and extract 85 consecutive cards from the middle of the tin containing details of male patients, and 95 from the middle of the tin containing details of female patients.

What might be the problem or biases, introduced by this method?

From the middle of the male tin the first six cards he might pick out are:

John MacEwan
Angus McTavish
James McTavish
Robert McTavish
Fred McTell
Brian Niall
George O'Connor
Patrick O'Malley

Dr Tipps begins to realize that names can 'cluster' into 'ethnic' and family groups.

Selection using this method is quite easy and convenient but it does not meet the requirements of the research question by giving a true cross-section of the patient population. This sample is unlikely to be sufficiently similar to the total population to enable him to generalize because it is not being selected from the whole patient population and every patient has not got an equal chance of selection. It is a sample of sorts but it is not a *representative sample*.

How can you ensure a representative sample?

For a study which measures the proportion of patients who smoke, Dr Tipps needs a sample that reproduces as accurately as possible the characteristics and qualities of the population on his list (which is the population he is studying). The intention is to use the results from the sample not just to draw implications for the sample itself but also to discuss the implications for the total population.

Random sampling is the most popular method for attempting to select a representative sample because it has the following qualities:

(1)   it overcomes selection bias by ensuring that each person in the population has an equal chance of being selected;

(2)   it should, if of sufficient size, adequately represent the population under study.

Question 2(3)

Dr Tipps then decides that his sample drawn as a group from his tins is not sufficiently representative of the population he wishes to study, for the reasons given above.

He decides to select every tenth card from each tin, starting with those aged 16 and working upwards through the age groups. Has this overcome all the objections with his previous method? Is this a truly random sample?

Well it is definitely better than the last sample, but it is not, strictly speaking, a random sample, unless the age–sex cards had all been filed in a random order. Since this defeats the object of an age–sex register, it is unlikely to be the case. This type of selection of one sample member whose selection is dependent on the selection of a previous one is called a *systematic sample*. In a small sample it will tend to produce a more even spread over the population list than does a simple random sample. In this instance a systematic sample is probably acceptable as it is unlikely that there is any constant 'pattern' in the ordering of patients. Selecting every thirteenth playing card from an unshuffled new pack would, of course, produce a very unrepresentative sample.

Undeterred, Dr Tipps decides he really wants a truly random sample, and so decides to use a table of random numbers (which he discovers can be found in the back of many statistics books). In the table he uses he finds that, starting at the top left corner, he must select the notes in the order: 3rd, 47th, 43rd, etc.

03	47	43	73	86		36	96	47	36	61
97	74	24	67	62		42	81	14	57	20
16	76	62	27	66		56	50	26	71	07
12	56	85	99	26						etc.

Alternatively he could have used some form of lottery, drawing the patient numbers out in a version of research workers' bingo. He could even have emptied the cards on his living room floor, mixed them all up thoroughly and trained his pet woodpecker, Woody, to pick out the required number. For obvious reasons, and since Woody was off-colour, he decided to use the tables of random numbers.

How big should the random sample be?

Should Dr Tipps select one patient in five; one in ten; or one in how many? The rule of thumb, given that many studies have severe practical limitations on them, is the bigger the better. However, it is no good selecting a large sample if there are not the facilities to gather or cope with the data when collected, nor a small one if it will not produce a valid result.

However, it is possible to calculate an idea of sample size required, by using some statistical techniques. The methods, and the exact formulae used will vary with the type of question being asked and the thing being measured, but they are based on the same principles. These and other statistical principles will be looked at in a later chapter, but it is worth spending a few minutes looking at their use in relation to sample size. (Don't worry if you do not follow the steps completely. You can always return to this later, especially when you have a practical problem of deciding on a sample size in reality; besides, by then you may have found a helpful local statistician to do the calculation for you.)

Dr Tipps wishes to know the proportion of his practice population aged over 16 who smoke. Let us assume the true figure is 34.5%.

If he were to take, say, five randomly chosen samples of 100 patients over 16, and asked them whether or not they smoked, he might find the following results:

	Smokers	Non-smokers
Sample 1	35	65
Sample 2	36	64
Sample 3	40	60
Sample 4	17	83
Sample 5	33	67

As can be seen, most results cluster around what we actually know to be the real population mean, but there are some outliers. If, by chance, sample 4 was drawn, then an invalid result would be produced to the question, 'What proportion of patients smoke?'

What we can say is that if he took a very large number of samples, say 50 samples of 100 patients each, then the mean of all these 50 sets of results would, to all intents and purposes, equal the mean of the population from which he took the sample. Some of the results would exactly equal the mean, some would be slightly more, some slightly less than the mean, and a few would be considerably more and a few considerably less than the mean. A graph drawn of these sets of results would appear as in Fig. 2.1.

As you can see, it is roughly bell-shaped, the ubiquitous *normal* curve about which doubtless you will have heard. At this stage the important points about the values which form this normal-curved shape are:

1.   Most of the results will be clustered around the 'true' mean—hence the 'bell' shape of their distribution. The exact shape of this bell can vary depending on how closely around the true mean value the results occur. A tall, peaked bell suggests that all the results were bunched around the mean value, whereas a flatter-shaped bell suggests that there was a wider spread of values.

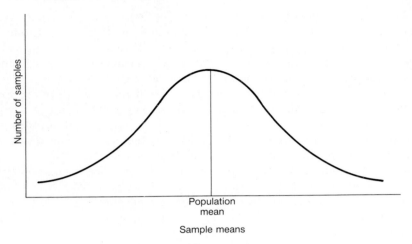

Fig. 2.1. The normal curve.

2.   There is a number which describes and summarizes the spread of this distribution and which can be calculated: it is known as the *standard error of the mean*. It is a fact that 95% of the means of each of the 50 samples taken will fall within 1.96 standard error distances from the true mean. Thus the standard error of a tall, peaked bell will be smaller than that of a flatter-shaped bell.

Why is all this important? Well, usually you only take one sample—after all, the whole idea of sampling is to cut down on the amount of time and effort. You need, therefore, to have some idea of this spread of the results (is the 'bell' likely to be peaked or flat), and as a consequence how likely your one result is to be near the true mean. The *standard error of the mean* can be used to give an indication of how likely the mean of your single sample (and therefore the representativeness of the sample) approximates the mean of the whole population.

In the case of Dr Tipps, where he wishes to know a proportion of a population with a certain characteristic, the formula by which one can derive the standard error (SE) is:

$$\text{SE} = \sqrt{\left(\frac{p\,(1-p)}{n}\right)}$$

where *p* is the proportion of the population with the characteristic being measured (in this case, smoking behaviour), *n* is the sample size, and where the population is known to be very large with respect to the size of the sample taken.

$$SE = \sqrt{\left(\frac{35 \times (100 - 35)}{100}\right)}$$
$$= 4.77$$

This means that he can state that there was a 95% chance that the true mean would fall within the range of the result found in this sample and 1.96 times the standard error: $35 \pm (1.96 \times 4.77)$. In other words, there is a 95% likelihood that the true proportion of his population who smoke lies between $35 \pm 9\%$, i.e. between 26 and 44%.

If his sample size had only been 10, the standard error would have been:

$$SE = \sqrt{\left(\frac{35 \times 65}{10}\right)}$$
$$= 15$$

In this case he would only have been able to say that there was a 95% chance that the population mean was between $35 \pm (1.96 \times 15)\%$, that is between 6 and 64%. As you can see, the 'accuracy' of his estimate for the population depends on the size of his sample. However, the extra accuracy to be gained by increasing the sample size tails off rapidly.

Exercise 2(2)

What would be the effect if his sample size had been:

(a)   500
(b)   1000

(You may need a calculator for the sums.) Answers are at the end of the chapter.

At this stage we are more interested in using the formula above to estimate the *size of sample* we require. As you can see, the formula can be rewritten in terms of *n* (the required size of the sample) as:

$$n = \frac{p(1 - p)}{(SE)^2}$$

A rough idea of the required size of a sample can be estimated if:

1.   an approximate result for the characteristic being measured can be found or guessed; and

2.   a decision can be made on the size of the standard error—that is, how accurate you require your sample to be in terms of how large or small a spread of results around the true mean you will be happy with.

For example, before taking his one sample, Phil Tipps knew that about 40% of the general population smoked. He also decided that he would like the result to be within about 10% of the true result, that is if the true result for his population was 36%, he wanted to be 95% certain that the result from his sample fell between $36 \pm 3.6\%$. He also knows that 95% of the samples will be within 1.96 standard errors of the mean. Therefore, for his project, he estimates that p will be 40 and that he needs the standard error to equal 1.8 (i.e. 3.6/1.96).

Substituting into the formula gives:

$$n = \frac{40 \times 60}{1.8 \times 1.8}$$

This would suggest that he would require a sample of around 750 to give him a result with the sort of accuracy he wishes.

As has been pointed out, the formula we have been using is only suitable when the characteristic being measured is a proportion. Other formulae based on exactly the same principles can be used for other measurements. These involve other statistical principles that we will meet later, and so we will return briefly to this subject then.

Therefore, in the case of the simple question 'How many smokers?', the method is quite straightforward as the aim is to get a large-enough sample to represent accurately the smoking behaviour of the background population.

That said, two further points emerge from this discussion of sample size. First, if you do not understand the maths don't worry. There are experts about who will help you with these technical issues. Not being able to grasp the meaning of the standard error need not prevent you from carrying out excellent research. Besides, for a lot of research this is not an issue: you either collect a total population sample, e.g. all your asthmatics, or as many as you can within the limits of your resources. There are, as we shall see in later chapters, ways of handling imperfect samples. However, because a sample size is not calculated for a lot of research, it does not mean that it should be dispensed with. Had the researchers in many studies completed this simple calculation, then their sample would have been seen as too small to obtain a significant result or—just as important—too large and therefore wasteful of time and resources.

Exercise 2(3)

1. Dr Tipps decides that he needs a more accurate result. He would like a 95% chance of the result being within 3% of the true mean. How large a sample would he need?

2. But this is the real world, he is a busy GP and he decides he can only afford the time to take a sample of 100. What predictions could he make about the accuracy of the result he will obtain from this sample in respect to the population?

Answers are given at the end of the chapter.

Before setting out with his postal questionnaire to ask what proportion of his patients smoke, Dr Tipps considers the other related question he wants answering.

Q. 'Who are the smokers?'

This question, as with the first, is aimed at gathering background information as it will be useful to find out not only the number of current smokers but also what their characteristics are. For example, if there is a particular interest in antenatal health education, it would be useful to know how many pregnant women smoke.

This question has a number of similar features to the first in that it is descriptive and is based on current patterns of behaviour, although it has two distinctive characteristics which have implications for the research design:

1. It distinguishes patients on more than one characteristic, i.e. smoking and pregnancy status.
2. It begins to examine the relationship or link between these two variables. For example, if you were to collect information about gender and smoking behaviour, you may find a higher proportion of male patients who are current smokers. In other words, there seems to be an *association* between gender and smoking. However, note that it only tells you if the variables are associated, and not if there is a causal relationship between the two.

The same sample might be used to answer the question, 'Who are the smokers?', as might be used to answer the question, 'What proportion smoke?'. As well as asking whether they smoke, they would be asked other questions, e.g. about their age, gender, marital status, so as to give further information about the smoking subgroup of patients.

Question 2(4)

Our Dr Tipps decides that he wants to make sure that each age band, as well as each sex, is adequately yet randomly represented in his sample, since he believes that one of the factors which is most strongly associated with smoking behaviour is age. How could he, with his age–sex register at home, allow for this?

Well, he has allowed for gender by selecting from his two separate tins; this ensures that men and women are fairly represented in the total sample. If he further wanted to ensure adequate representation of each age band, he could 'group' his ages, as if in separate tins, before sampling from them. Thus, first he could calculate the number of patients within each band, e.g. those aged 16–25, 26–35, 36–45, etc.; then he would calculate the numbers required for his 10% sample; and then, by using the table of random numbers, he would select an appropriate random sample from each of these age strata within each sex. This is a *stratified random sample*. In this case it would be stratified for age and sex.

For example, if Dr Tipps is particularly concerned about smoking among under-25s he may wish to stratify by age to ensure their adequate representation in the sample. First he would calculate the number of 16–25-year-olds among men and women in the practice. Dr Tipps finds that this age group account for almost exactly 15% of both men and women. If he used random sampling, he would therefore expect to obtain 27 individuals from this group in his overall sample of 190 patients. However, he may, by chance, only get 24 or even 20 (though he may of course get more). By age stratifying his sample into under- and over-25 he can then randomly choose 27 and 163 cases from each group, so ensuring correct representation of his under-25s.

Dr Tipps could also take this logic further. He might decide that 27 is rather a small group to analyse, particularly when split into men and women. He might therefore 'weight' this under-25 sample by a factor of, say, four, thereby choosing 108 instead of 27 patients. He could always 'reconstitute' his original representative sample by dividing the under-25s by four and adding them back in.

In summary, stratification is the process of dividing the sample population into strata prior to sampling so as to increase population and representativeness, especially of limited sample sizes. Usually, factors chosen for stratification are those felt to be closely related to the subject of the survey, although selection of factors will also depend upon availability of information. For example, although social class is also likely to be strongly associated with cigarette smoking, it may be impossible to stratify for it as there may be no information on social class in an age–sex register.

Exercise 2(4)

1.   You are concerned that some patients have difficulty in getting up the steep driveway to your surgery. You decide to find out who they are by means of a questionnaire. Who would you send it to?
(a)   A random sample of all your patients.
(b)   A random sample of those attending this month.
(c)   An age-stratified sample of patients of all your patients.
(d)   An age-stratified sample of patients who consult this month.
(e)   All those who your receptionists note have had difficulty with the driveway.

2.   You wonder if your patients would like to read their own notes. You design a questionnaire. Who would you send it to?
(a)   A random sample of all your patients?
(b)   A random sample of all your patients aged over 16.
(c)   A random sample of all your patients who can read.
(d)   A random sample of all the patients who see you in the next week.
(e)   A random sample of your most responsible patients.

3.   You wonder if the time you spend counselling your patients is having any effect. You decide to allocate randomly to counselling and non-counselling groups and count the number of subsequent consultations as a measure of success. Who would you enter into the study?

(a)   All the patients you see in a week.
(b)   All the patients with psychosocial problems you see in a week.
(c)   A random sample of all your patients.
(d)   Any patient you see with blue eyes.
(e)   Any patient you see with a birthday on an odd day of the month.

Suggested answers are at the end of the chapter.

Having found out how many smokers there are and who they are, the next stage of Dr Tipps's research is to look at how the doctor can influence smoking behaviour.

Q   'Does the advice that I give to cigarette smokers actually change their awareness, their attitudes, or their smoking behaviour?

The aim of this research question is to evaluate the effect of the doctor's intervention. What are the differences between this question and the first two?

The major difference is that this third question is not just concerned with identifying a link or an association between two variables, but whether one variable is causally related to the other. In this case the aim is to see whether, amongst all of the possible influences on cigarette smoking, the intervention by the doctor through giving advice has any impact. In other words, does the advice given by the doctor actually *cause* a change in the awareness, attitudes, or behaviour of the patient?

Before Dr Tipps can decide on the appropriate design, it is important to look at what is meant by a causal influence, as the question of causality and correlation is central to most research studies.

Does employment cause ill-health?
Is sugar intake related to diabetes?
Is asbestos linked with cancer?
Does stress cause heart attacks?
Is tennis correlated with baldness?

Each of these examples involves two variables held in some sort of relationship to one another: 'caused', 'linked', 'related', 'correlated', etc. What do these words actually mean? They are all variations on 'cause', which is the fundamental link which any researcher is chasing, though some of them express the notion of cause in a very weak sort of way.

What are the stages we must go through before we can say that something causes something else?

There are three conditions which must be fulfilled before one can strongly suggest that A causes B:

(1)   the temporal sequence must be right with A preceding B in time;

(2)   there must be a correlation between the variables, such that as A varies so B varies also; and

(3)   there must be no significant 'third' variable. If a third variable (confounding factor) exists, which affects both A and B, then the observed relationship between the latter might be 'spurious'.

Let us look at this third condition in a little more detail. All so-called causal relationships are, in fact, provisional and can be constantly subjected to challenge by suggesting other variables which explain the observed correlation. Thus, for example, the 'causal' connection:

$$\text{smoking} \rightarrow \text{IHD}$$

may really be:

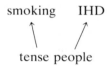

Thus, an important component of research is to take existing 'known' relationships, which are seen as causal in nature, and suggest alternative explanations of why the two (or more) variables seem to be related. Thinking of 'alternative explanations' is very important. Most 'great science' is not discovering new things but finding better explanations for known phenomena. Try it! When reading or listening to a research paper you come across a supposed relationship between two or more variables think, 'How else might this relationship be explained?' There are *always* alternatives; most are probably fanciful, cosmic rays, men from Mars, MI5 blunders, but occasionally you will come across an interesting alternative. The next stage is how to express this as a researchable question (back to Chapter 1), and then how to devise an appropriate design.

Exercise 2(5)

Suggest some alternative hypotheses for the following supposed 'causal' relationships:

(a)   high blood sugar and retinopathy;
(b)   TB bacillus and tuberculosis;
(c)   smoking and gastric ulcer;
(d)   stress and ulcerative colitis;
(e)   promiscuity and cervical cancer;
(f)   snoring and CHD.

Suggested answers are at the end of the chapter.

Let's continue with Dr Tipps's study of health education and consider the range of designs which might be available for assessing the impact of advice. In each case the design must enable the question to be answered and help rule out some of the more obvious alternative explanations. Three possible designs are:

(1)   one group after information;

(2)   two groups after information;

(3)   two groups before and after information.

One group after information

The first design is the most simple and would involve collecting information from smokers *after* they had received advice from their doctors. Let us assume that smoking declined: would that confirm the hypothesis that the advice was effective? (That is, is there an alternative explanation?)

It is possible that something else happened at the same time (e.g. a national anti-smoking campaign) which produced the observed affect. We need to allow for such extraneous factors—technically, *control* for them. But how can you do this without knowing what they are? The most straightforward way is to have a *control group* which will experience everything, including any other health educational campaign, except the doctor's advice.

Two groups after information

The second design fulfils this condition, in that it compares a group that did not receive any advice with one that did. The two groups are then asked about their smoking practices over the last year or so. If it is found that the 'advice' group (the intervention group) report a steeper decline in smoking than the control group, is it then possible to conclude that the advice is effective? A qualified 'yes', because there are still some caveats. The interpretation of the results depends on both how the two groups were selected and the reliability of retrospective reporting of smoking.

The selection of groups

The aim of the study design is to attempt to identify two groups identical in every way apart from the fact that one will receive advice and the other will not. Thus the method of selection of the two groups is crucial so as to minimize any bias.

Two methods are available:

● random allocation;
● matched control groups.

Random allocation means that the group, intervention, or control, to which a case is assigned for study is determined by chance, so that each person who enters the study has the same chance of being in either group. Thus, in the study of giving advice about cigarette smoking, each patient who is a current smoker would be randomly allocated, using random numbers, to the control or to the experimental groups. The concept of randomness was discussed briefly in the previous section and it will become clear that by using random allocation the two groups selected should be similar in terms of most characteristics, apart from the fact that one group received advice and the other did not.

Matched control groups have certain similarities to stratified sampling, in that some factors are deliberately manipulated rather than being left to chance as in randomization. Patients in the intervention and the control groups are matched by factors such as age, social class, educational background, and other factors with which it is known that cigarette smoking varies, thus producing what is called a *case control study*. Some of the data on which to base the matching could be collected in answer to the earlier question of 'Who smokes?'

One difficulty with matching is that the factors to match for are not always clear, and it may only be possible to match for some, and not all, the contaminating factors.

A second problem is that if, say, five or six factors are being controlled for, it may be difficult to find matching pairs. A simpler but less precise technique is to match the two groups for the variables separately, not in combination. In principle, therefore, six middle-class married men and six working-class unmarried men in the sample could be 'matched' by six working-class married men and six middle-class unmarried men in the control group—though, in practice, variables do get more mixed up than this.

Clearly, if random allocation to the intervention and control groups were chosen, it would have to take place prior to the doctor giving advice. If the study is a *retrospective* one, investigating the effect of an intervention which has already taken place, (for example, comparing current respiratory illness in a group which did and did not receive antibiotics in childhood), then random allocation is impossible and the case control study comes into its own.

Retrospective data

Because the research is concerned with the possible causal influence of the advice (the intervention variable) on cigarette smoking (the outcome variable), it should be helpful to have a design which:

- shows changes in smoking behaviour over time;
- can identify the relationships between these changes and the advice given by the doctor.

The aim would be to compare changes in smoking during a time period, starting sometime before and finishing some time after the doctor gave the advice. This would also apply to the control group. In the case of the two-group design, however, you would have to rely on smokers' reports of their current behaviour and their past behaviour, gathered through information collected after the advice was given.

This gathering of data through retrospective reports is a popular method for trying to find out about changes over time and the factors that influence them. However, retrospective reporting is fraught with problems associated with:

- weakness in memory recall;
- current experience and behaviour colouring reports of past behaviour;
- reports influenced by what 'ought' to have occurred.

Each of these problems is important, although the first two could equally apply to both advice and control groups. However, the third problem may apply particularly to the advice group who may tailor their reports of the degree of change of smoking behaviour to what they feel the doctor wanted to happen.

Two groups before and after information

The third design overcomes the problem of retrospective reports and their inherent biases. This design is what is called a 'before and after design', where the behaviour in question is measured both some time before and after the intervention. This before and after design would also have to be used in the control group or comparison groups. This would ensure that changes in behaviour found to be associated with the intervention did not reflect changes in behaviour which had occurred concurrently, perhaps generated by other influences, such as a national campaign aimed at changing smoking habits, or large increases in the price of cigarettes. This idea of following up the same group (cohort) of people to identify changes in behaviour or other factors is described as a *cohort* or *longitudinal* design, in contrast to the measurement at one point in time, which is called a *cross-sectional* design.

The best design to test the proposition, then, would be a two-group before and after design. This design can be refined in a number of different ways to cope with other issues. For example, if both groups were to be interviewed about their cigarette smoking before and after, you may be concerned about the effect of the interview on their behaviour. The interview may have the effect of raising awareness and encouraging modification in smoking behaviour. Thus, a third group would need to be added which not only did not receive advice but also had a brief form to complete rather than a questionnaire through interview.

It should be clear from the above discussion that in general practice, choice of research design has to be pragmatic. There might be an 'ideal' design, but often practical constraints involve choosing another. However, this does not mean that the more 'classical' formal research designs, as found for example in epidemiology, are not used in general practice; indeed we have covered several of the more common ones above. These have included the use of experimental designs such as randomized or case control studies and longitudinal designs aimed at measuring changes over time.

Exercise 2(6)

Identify the appropriate research *design* for answering the following questions:

(a)   Do men have higher consultation rates than women?
(b)   Do longer consultations increase levels of patient satisfaction?
(c)   Are working-class patients more likely to be dissatisfied with their doctors than middle-class patients?
(d)   What proportion of the patients on your list are heavy drinkers?
(e)   Do shorter consultations lead to higher prescribing?

Suggested answers are given at the end of the chapter.

The results of the evaluation may show that the advice given by the doctor has had a major impact or perhaps only a modest impact. However, what if it had no effect at all, or at least no measurable effect? The next question would be to ask why it had no effect:

Q.   Why does my advice have this impact?

This question is trying to investigate the relationship between variables, but not just in a statistical sense, as it is concerned with understanding the *nature* of the relationship between what the doctor said and how the patient responded. It would seem better in this particular case to use a qualitative approach.

WHAT IS QUALITATIVE RESEARCH?

Qualitative research is usually contrasted with quantitative research. The latter is concerned with counting, with reducing phenomena to numbers. But there are many phenomena, it is argued, which cannot be captured in a number, or at least are destroyed by any attempt to do so. Imagine asking your patients how they feel today and one says 'I feel very grey today'. Perhaps that statement could be reduced to a number, but might it not be possible to keep and analyse the statement in that form? This is the basis of qualitative research, which, as its name suggests, collects and analyses qualitative data.

One of the major criticisms levelled at much quantitative research is that it tends to restrict the sorts of answers that can be obtained. The question 'Have you come to the doctor today because you are ill or because you want him to sign a passport form?' does not allow space for the patient who wants to catch up on last year's *Country Life* in the waiting room. The question 'Why have you come to the doctor today?' would pick this up, as well as a hundred other idiosyncratic reasons. Analysing this data is, as we shall see, difficult (the quantitative study's closed question is a doddle in comparison), but at least it better captures the real reasons for attendance. For this reason qualitative studies are often used to answer 'why' questions. The emphasis is on an intensive investigation of a small number of cases or settings. Also, a qualitative approach can be used in an exploratory way to establish the sorts of questions it would be most appropriate to ask in a quantitative questionnaire-based survey, so that the possible answers provided for a question bear a closer relationship to the respondents' real range of views.

A qualitative approach could be used in the investigation of why GP advice about smoking is ineffective, and could begin with interviews of a small group of smokers who received advice but did not report any change in behaviour. In this type of investigation the research design is of little importance as no claims are being made about the representativeness of the sample nor are attempts being made to control for extraneous factors. The emphasis is on understanding the nature of the relationship between variables, and identifying the processes which shape that relationship. In this way, it might be found that the no-change group received half-hearted advice, or perhaps did not appear to understand the terms the doctor used.

One of the basic assumptions behind this type of interviewing is that people are not empty vessels but have their own complex belief-systems supplied by their culture and influenced by their experiences. Thus any understanding of their behaviour and their reasons for their behaviour should begin by examining the sets of beliefs, rules, and meanings, which govern their daily lives. An understanding of smoking behaviour and the impact of doctors' advice will require an investigation of patients' beliefs about smoking, and its relationship to health and to the meaning of the advice given by the doctor.

The methods adopted should aim to elicit the beliefs and feelings of the smoker without being influenced by the assumptions and values of the researcher. The most popular method for this approach is unstructured interviewing using tape-recorders. This involves the interviewer having a list of topics or general questions about which the interviewee is invited to express his or her own views. The tape-recorded interview is transcribed word for word and the transcripts are subsequently analysed (see Chapter 4 on data collection).

The method of sampling that could be used in this case would be *quota sampling*. Quota sampling makes no pretence at randomness, it simply means that the interviewer selects sufficient cases with the desired charac- teristics (e.g. women, elderly, bald men, etc.) to make up the sample size. Because the emphasis is on examining the different types of relationships, it is important to choose, quite deliberately, a wide range of respondents.

The major weakness with quota sampling is that it is non-random and this makes it difficult, if not impossible, to estimate how representative the samples are of the population. The major advantage of quota sampling is that it is economical and time-saving and is particularly useful in explora- tory research using a qualitative methodology.

SUMMARY

In this chapter we have looked at the questions that need to be thought about when deciding on a research design for a study. Specifically, we have shown how the adoption of a certain type of design will depend upon the nature of the research question being examined.

SUGGESTED TASKS

Select some articles from medical journals and for each:

1. identify the research question being asked;
2. identify the research design chosen;
3. think of alternative designs;
4. decide whether your alternatives would have been constrained on ethical grounds or by cost.

ANSWERS TO EXERCISES

Exercise 2(1)

1. *Telephone directory*. The main advantage of the telephone directory is that it is easily accessible, although its major disadvantage is that it will be unrepresentative. While a large majority of the population do have their own telephones, the proportion who do not will be mainly those who cannot afford to.

2. *Electoral register*. An electoral register can be obtained from a public library. It is compiled every October and published the following spring. It lists, within each Polling district, all those entitled to vote (aged 18 or over). It is probably the most convenient method for identifying a representative sample of the general population. The vast majority of

people who are eligible to register actually do (96%), although it does not represent people under 18 and non-British subjects. There is also a problem with the proportion of people who move (8% per year) and how to trace them for interview.

3. *Rating records*. The rating record can be obtained from local authorities (contact the Valuation Officer). The major role of the rating records is to sample housing properties. It has no advantages over the electoral register for gaining a sample of individuals or households, in that it will only represent those paying rates. There are doubts also about how up-to-date the records are. At the time of writing it is unclear how available or accurate poll-tax records will be, although they are likely to be similar to the electoral register.

Exercise 2(2)

1. A sample of 500:

$$\text{SE} = \sqrt{\left(\frac{35 \times 65}{500}\right)}$$
$$= 2.1$$

Therefore the percentage of smokers was 95% certain of being between 31 and 39% [i.e. $35 \pm (1.96 \times 2.1)$].

2. A sample of 100:

$$\text{SE} = \sqrt{\left(\frac{35 \times 65}{1000}\right)}$$
$$= 1.5$$

Therefore the percentage of smokers was 95% certain of being between 32 and 37% [i.e. $35 \pm (1.96 \times 1.5)$].

As you can see, doubling the sample size when it already involves fairly large numbers has a smaller effect on the precision of the answer obtained.

Exercise 2(3)

1. Dr Tipps wants the answer to be more precise, he would like it to be within 3% of the real value. He assumes again that the true mean is around 40%, and therefore he would like to be 95% certain that his result would be within 3% of this, that is that the SE would be 1.2/1.96, i.e. 0.6.

Substituting into the formula:

$$n = \frac{40(100 - 40)}{0.6 \times 0.6}$$
$$= 6666$$

Therefore in order to be 95% certain that his result was within 3% of the true mean, he would need to take a sample of about 6500.

2. He can only take a sample of 100. Again using his estimate of the result being around 40%, he finds:

$$SE\ (p) = \sqrt{\left(\frac{40 \times (100 - 40)}{100}\right)}$$
$$= 4.89$$

He therefore knows that the true proportion of smokers in his population is 95% likely to be within 9.5% of the mean he obtains from his sample.

Exercise 2(4)

1. (a) This would work but it is a big hammer to crack a small nut. Moreover, the numbers having difficulty with the driveway are likely to be small in the sample.

(b) Some improvement on the above, at least you restrict the sample to those who consult; those who don't consult cannot have trouble with the driveway (unless they do not consult because they cannot make it up the drive).

(c) and (d) Age stratification seems sensible: numbers having difficulty are likely to be few and are more likely to be elderly, so this, especially (d), should ensure that the main 'at risk' group is properly represented in your sample.

(e) Why bother with the questionnaire? You could simply ask your receptionist. The problem is that your receptionist might miss some people—in which case a sample derived from them would be inappropriate.

2. (a), (b), (c) These are all possibilities. Presumably you would want to restrict it to adults and to those who can read but you are unlikely to have data on the latter. Thus sample (b) would seem the best of the three.

(d) Consulters are not representative of all your patients so this sample is 'biased'. However, it may be that the question of reading notes is more appropriate for consulters, who might have both the wish and the opportunity to read their notes. If you accept this assumption, this would be the best sample.

(e) Well this is one way of fixing it. You could choose as 'responsible' all those patients who agree with your views; the result will then be to your liking. Politically shrewd—but is it research?

3.   (a)   This depends on whether you think counselling might benefit all your patients who consult. If you think it will, this would be the one to go for.

(b)   More realistically you might want to start only with those who might be said to 'need' counselling.

(c)   But how can the non-consulters receive the treatment or non-treatment? However, you could use your total patient population to 'mark' out those who will and those who will not receive counselling if they do consult. If your sample is truly random and your population large enough, you should have allocated those who consult with emotional problems next week into two equally sized groups.

(d)   This is one way of getting a sample but only 'safe' if blue eyes are totally unconnected with having emotional difficulties or being responsive to counselling. You probably cannot make these assumptions, particularly if your practice contains large ethnic groups.

(e)   Similar to (d), but it is less likely that birth date is related to illness or treatment. In fact this is probably a reasonable way of obtaining a 50% sample or, by using odd and even birth dates, of randomized patients between two groups.

Exercise 2(5)

1.   Arteriopathy might cause retinopathy and also affect the pancreas to interfere with insulin production, hence increasing blood sugar.

2.   An 'autoimmune response' might generate a tuberculous-like lesion, e.g. Crohns, and also allow the bacillus entry to the body if contact is made: hence they would tend to occur together as in gastrointestinal tuberculosis.

3.   Anxious people might be both more likely to smoke and more likely to get a gastric ulcer.

4.   Stress may be a response in people genetically predisposed; they might also be genetically predisposed to ulcerative colitis. Hence the two would be more likely to occur together.

5.   Women with unhappy childhoods might be more likely to be promiscuous; the unhappiness might also—through an unknown mechanism—make them more at risk for developing cervical cancer.

6.   Impaired respiratory function might produce snoring as well as placing extra effort on the heart.

These are only suggestions—some of them fairly pathetic—and you might have better ones. The important point to stress is the possibility of constantly searching for alternatives for both speculative and even 'established' truths.

Exercise 2(6)

(a) and (c)   Bivariate analysis with cross-sectional design.

(b) and (e)   Before-and-after design with controls.

(d)   Descriptive cross-sectional designs.

3 Measuring things

This chapter examines how you will go about measuring the things that you have decided need measuring in your research design.

In her clinical work, Dr Melanie Warmhands has observed that the relationships in the families of asthmatic children do not seem very good. How should she go about exploring this question? Let us briefly summarize the process covered so far.

First, as argued in Chapter 1, the hunch must be refined into a *researchable hypothesis*. This might be:

The relationships between the parents of an asthmatic child are of poor quality.

Secondly, as presented in Chapter 2, an appropriate *research design* must be chosen for the project. Obviously, this must involve examining the relationships between parents of asthmatic children to see if they are indeed of poor quality.

How will Dr Warmhands choose her sample?

Question 3(1)

Below are four different ways of getting a sample. Score each of these from 1 (worst) to 5 (best) for two qualities: ideal suitability and practical suitability.

(a) picking out the next 20 known asthmatic children who present (sample A);
(b) questioning and examining all the children who present with asthma until 20 cases have accumulated (sample B);
(c) randomly select case notes of children until there are 20 with a history of asthma (sample C);
(d) randomly select case notes of children, visit them and examine for asthma, until there are 20 cases (sample D).

Three of these methods of sampling have a bias, that is they involve selecting for criteria other than asthma:

(a) Sample A is a selection of children:
● with asthma;
● who are attenders;
● who are known to the GP;

(b) Sample B is a selection of children:
● with asthma;
● who are attenders.

(c)   Sample C is a selection of children:
● with asthma;
● who are known to the GP.

(d)   Sample D is a selection of children:
● with asthma (open to bias in the representativeness of the case notes).

Should sample D therefore be chosen? There are other considerations, chief of which is practicality. Sample D is only obtained after considerable time and energy. In contrast, sample A, which is the most biased, is the most easily obtained. What relative weights should be given to these two factors of bias and practicality?

The answer has to involve consideration of the research question: if necessary it might have to be revised. The hypothesis as stated would suggest that sample D is the best because the question tries to make a general statement about parents of *all* asthmatics. On the other hand, the question evolved from a clinical observation which presumably only involved known asthmatics and attenders. In this sense there is some justification in clarifying the research hypothesis:

The relationships between the parents of known asthmatic children who consult their GP are of poor quality.

This hypothesis would allow the use of sample A; however, by narrowing the focus some other difficulties have been introduced:

● The research question is not as wide as it was and there will be little to conclude about non-attending asthmatics (although if the hypothesis was confirmed, it would be possible to go on to spread the net wider in a follow-up study).
● The original question suggested some relationship between asthma in a child and parental dynamics, perhaps that poor parental relationships somehow 'produced' asthma in their child. If a relationship between asthma and parental dynamics was found in this particular sample, a very plausible alternative explanation would have to be considered, namely that poor parental relationships cause attendance or cause their child to be brought for diagnosis. Some of this threat to the interpretation of the findings can be allowed for in the other important element of research design, namely a control group. In addition, there is clearly a need for a control group to measure 'poor quality' because this obviously implies 'poorer quality than other parental relationships'. (If other relationships are not checked, it could be that all the parents on a GP's list have similar poor relationships and therefore asthma is not unusual in this respect.)

Dr Warmhands chooses sample A. She obtains 20 children for her sample. Which of the following would be a suitable control group?

(a)   20 other children seen in the period, randomly selected;
(b)   20 other children seen in the period, with the same ages and sexes of the asthmatic sample, i.e. matched;
(c)   20 other children seen in the period, with chronic eczema.

Each of these control groups has its merits:

• A random sample as in (a) would go some way to allow for the characteristics of sample A which might confuse the answer to the question. Say, for example, that poor parental dynamics did not affect asthma but rather increased the likelihood of a surgery attendance; a relationship would then be found between asthmatics attending surgery and parental relationships because asthmatics also happen to be attenders. If there was a control group of random attenders, these should also show poor parental relationships. Therefore, it would be possible to conclude from this that the finding among the asthmatics was a *spurious* one, unrelated to asthma. On the other hand, if there was a difference between asthmatics and controls it would tend to support the view that it is the asthma itself which is the significant factor.

• While a random sample has clear advantages as a control group, in practice quite large numbers might be necessary to be sure that extraneous factors have been properly randomized. For example, just by chance, the control group might have an average age higher than the asthmatic group, thus any observed difference in parental relationships might reflect this fact rather than the asthma. With small numbers, as in sample A, a matched control group removes some of the biases which might confound the comparisons. Thus matching for age and sex ensures that these factors cannot be used to explain any differences between the asthmatic children and the control group, because they are both exactly the same with regard these variables.

• Control group (c) is another form of matching. Here the logic is to exclude factors from the study which might contaminate the role of asthma. Thus it is possible that poor parental interrelationship in asthmatics and attendance rates are somehow related, not to the asthma itself but simply to having a chronic illness. Hence by controlling for other chronic illnesses, or a specific one, any difference between the relationships in the two groups is more likely to be linked to asthma itself.

After due consideration of the above issues Dr Warmhands chooses control group (c). She now has a prospective matched control group design with which to test her hypothesis; now, on to measuring things.

MEASUREMENT

In this study Dr Warmhands has to decide which attributes she is going to measure and what sort of 'ruler' she is going to use. The technical term for the device with which she will measure is an 'instrument'.

First, what does she need to measure? There would seem to be at least six different keywords contained in the research question:

(a)   children;

(b)   attendance;

(c)   asthma;

(d)   eczema;

(e)   parent;

(f)   interpersonal relationship;

(g)   other 'control' variables.

Each of these 'things' is a 'variable' because it can be expected to vary. In addition, they all have a certain abstract quality about them because at the moment they are simply words: we might be able to guess what they mean, but for the research we shall have to be very precise about how we define them.

Each of these words is a *concept*. They are concepts because they involve an idea or quality which is fairly abstract. We cannot physically get hold of these qualities, though if we knew how to define or measure them then we should be able at least to identify them. In short, we need some measure or *indicator* of the quality which we are interested in. This process, of devising indicators for concepts, is known as *operationalization* and is the main concern of the rest of this chapter.

How does Dr Warmhands operationalize the variable list above? Let's take each in turn.

(1)   Children
We all know what children are in everyday terms, but let us suspend that knowledge for a moment while we go through the process of how we measure 'children' in a research project.

What ideas do we start with about children? We can agree that children are small, and playful, and that they lack the intellectual grasp of an adult. How, therefore, do we measure whether someone who consults with us is a child or not? There are various possibilities given the above ideas on what a child is:

(a)   establish their height: those below 5 feet are children;

(b)   provide with coloured bricks and see if they play: if they do, they are children;

(c)   establish their intellectual age: if it is less than 10, they are children;

(d)   ask their chronological age: if it is less than 12, they are children.

Which instrument is chosen will depend on what is meant by children *in the context of this study*. In a psychiatric study we might look for child-like intellectual activities in adults, but in this research there is a clear understanding that children are differentiated by the chronological age. This still leaves open the cut-off point. At what age does Dr Warmhands want children to be eligible to enter her sample and at what age do they become too old? These decisions are fairly arbitrary. She decides that she is really only interested in asthma in schoolchildren and she therefore selects the ages of 5 and 15 as the bottom and top delimiters. Thus she concludes:

A child, in the context of this study, is anyone over the age of 4 and under the age of 16 at the time of being seen. Furthermore their quality of 'childness' will be measured by using a scale based on their age, i.e. from 5 to 15, which will be obtained by asking them how old they are.

The example of measuring a child is somewhat trivial but it illustrates both the logic of measurement and the fact that even very familiar things need to be clearly defined *before* starting to collect data. In summary, then, there is a *concept*, a child, which can be *operationalized* by using the response to the question 'How old are you?' as an *indicator*.

Exercise 3(1)

Concepts and indicators. Match the following *concepts* to the appropriate *indicators*.

income	aged over 65
elderly	presence of a vagina
women	sphygmomanometer reading
stress	monthly net salary
chronic illness	heart rate
GP workload	reported gender
referral rate	galvanic skin resistance
blood pressure	length of surgeries
	on disability register
	reports long-standing illness
	number of patients seen
	patients sent to OP

Suggested answers are given at the end of the chapter.

You may notice that taken *in isolation* what is a concept and what is an indicator are rather arbitrary. Thus 'heart rate' is an indicator of 'stress' but, equally, heart rate could be treated as a concept and operationalized as, say, pulse rate in the radial artery. The key difference between the two is therefore their relative positions:

- concepts are always more abstract than indicators, indicators more empirical than concepts;
- concepts are drawn from the hypothesis in question, indicators describe practical measurement procedures.

Exercise 3(2)

Operationalize the following hypotheses:

(a)   older people are more likely to be diabetic;
(b)   your concentration tends to lapse towards the end of a surgery;
(c)   you have more elderly patients on your list than your partners;
(d)   patients with stress in their lives consult more frequently;
(e)   a patient's hand movement while describing an anginal pain is very characteristic.

Remember: For each you could, if you wish, plan out a research design. In addition, you should list the concepts you wish to measure and against each one list one or more possible indicators.

Suggested answers are given at the end of the chapter.

Reliability and validity

The instrument chosen to measure whether or not the patient is a child or not is basically the question 'How old are you?' The answer identifies whether or not this is a child for the purposes of the study and what 'childness' qualities they have. Having operationalized 'child' there are two important questions that need to be asked of the instrument:

(a)   Is it reliable?
(b)   Is it valid?

Reliability

Reliability is a technical term. It refers to whether or not an instrument gives consistent results. A ruler is reliable because successive measurements of the same length would produce the same result. Is the question 'How old are you?' reliable? Yes, it is highly unlikely that people's responses will vary over a period of time (unless they have had birthdays). It may, however, be unreliable if applied to very small children or to a preliterate society in which chronological age is simply a guess.

Validity

Validity refers to whether the instrument measures what it purports to measure. A way of measuring may be reliable yet still be invalid. Thus, while readings from a sphygmomanometer may be consistent, they may also be mistakenly consistent (if the machine is miscalibrated).

For the moment there is a need to establish how valid the question 'How old are you?' is, as a means of measuring the chronological age of the child.

There are various different ways of establishing the validity of an instrument: the most basic are face validity and convergent validity.

Face validity. We can argue that the instrument ('How old are you?') is valid because it seems obvious that this question will establish a correct answer. This form of validity is referred to as *face validity* or *logical validity* because 'on the face of it' it seems correct.

Much of measurement in medicine relies on face validity. There is often a general consensus that certain 'instruments' actually measure what they purport to measure (hence the synonymous term of *consensus validity*). Thus, in clinical practice a high blood sugar indicates diabetes; raised cardiac enzymes, a myocardial infarction; pain in the right iliac fossa, appendicitis; etc. And, of course, the same thing goes for research when measurement often seems unproblematic.

The problem with this approach is that the instrument may be invalid or a better one may be overlooked. Exacerbation of abdominal pain on walking is, for example, probably a better indicator of appendicitis than localization to the RIF (according to researchers who have studied the validity of various indicators of appendicitis). This does not mean that face validity is an unsuitable way of assessing the value of an indicator, in many situations it will be quite appropriate. The message is that face validity is only one way of doing it—and a fairly low-level way at that—and you might like to consider alternatives; but above all you need to be aware of the assumptions behind face validity if you use it as the basis of your measurement.

Convergent validity. Face validity is in many ways the weakest way of establishing validity because it is clearly open to the idiosyncracies of the researcher to decide what is 'obvious'. Perhaps children lie about their age? How can it be established that a question on their age gives a truthful answer? The simplest means is to seek corroboration: we might ask to see their birth certificate, check their notes, ask their parents, etc. Again we cannot be absolutely sure, but if all these indicators provide exactly the same answer we can feel reasonably confident that our initial instrument, namely a question to the child, is valid.

This form of corroboration is called *convergent validity*, in that different measures all 'converge' to support one another. In addition, convergent validity can be divided into two types: *concurrent* in which the corroborative measure is established at the same time, or it may be *predictive* in which the supporting data is gathered sometime in the future.

The surgeon usually looks for additional indicators of appendicitis beyond RIF pain before making the diagnosis; physicians will use an ECG recording to support the implications of raised cardiac enzymes; etc. Does a high blood sugar indicate diabetes? Well it might have predictive validity if it were established that patients with high blood sugar had a greater chance of developing retinopathy. And so on. In effect, a disease or diagnostic category is simply a word given to a clustering of indicators.

Exercise 3(3)

Professor Teasmade, the well-known GP and ornithologist, has just presented his latest research to a typically uncritical and ingratiating group of acolytes. Alert to the problems of the validity of his measures—and anxious to establish your reputation as a fast young blade—you publicly challenge him: what type of validity does he use in his replies?

Q.1.   How do you know you measured blood pressure accurately?
A.   My sphygmomanometer is recalibrated every six months.
Q.2.   How do you know patients' self-reporting was a valid measure of chronic illness?
A.   Because I checked them with my own impeccable clinical records.
Q.3.   How do you know that you were able to distinguish severe angina from your series of chest pains?
A.   Most of them had admissions for myocardial infarction the following year—that's pretty serious! (laughter)
Q.4.   How do you know that you did not forget to record any patients when you calculated your consultation rate?
A.   Because my devoted receptionist also kept a record.
Q.5.   How did you establish which of your patients had a high stress level? (cries of "sit down!")
A.   It was fairly obvious to a person of my skill and experience. (applause)

Suggested answers are given at the end of the chapter.

(2)   Attendance

The hypothesis requires the sample to be drawn from children who see the doctor. How is Dr Warmhands to accomplish this? Again, it is partly a definitional exercise because as long as attendance is defined and measured the same way for both asthmatic children and controls then they should be comparable. Even so, defining 'attendance' is not as easy as it might at first seem.

Question 3(2)

Which of the following children would be eligible for inclusion in a sample of *attenders*?

An asthmatic child:

(a) who is brought in with a cough;
(b) who accompanies its mother who has booked the consultation for herself;
(c) who comes to collect a repeat prescription for his/her parent;
(d) whom you visit at home to investigate an abdominal pain;
(e) whom you chance to meet in the local supermarket;
(f) whom you visit in hospital following his/her emergency admission.

There are in fact no right or wrong answers. The operationalization of 'attendance' can be fairly arbitrary so long as it is consistent. Thus, Dr Warmhands might decide:

● attendance is a consultation with the child in the surgery.

Is it reliable? So long as the decision is consistent. Is it valid? The indicator has face validity.

(3) Asthma
How will asthma be measured? Dr Warmhands cannot, as in 'attendance' say that asthma is what she says it is, because there are accepted outside definitions of asthma which must act as her standard.

What is asthma? How is it defined clinically? A search of the literature will reveal that there is no generally accepted standard diagnostic criterion which can simply be taken off the shelf. There are many ways of defining asthma and as many controversies about what exactly it is. How should Dr Warmhands go about choosing?

She could go back to the original clinical observation. What was meant by asthma in that observation? Can it be reproduced in a reliable way? Alternatively she could look to other researchers who have operationalized it and use their approach. What about taking reduced peak-flow as an indicator?

● Is it practical and easy? Yes, it is a simple, cheap, and straightforward technique which should be easy to carry out for 5—15-year-olds.
● Is it reliable? There may be an existing literature on this, which could be checked. Alternatively she could try it herself—clinically she may already be doing so by making three measures and choosing the 'best'. For research, however, we are interested in the relative similarities of the readings. If, after an initial practice, readings seem reasonably consistent, we can conclude that the technique is reliable.
● Is it valid? Does a low peak-flow indicate asthma? This is a question with several answers. First, it could be that a definition of asthma will include low peak-flow. Secondly, there may already be a literature on the validity of peak flow as an indicator of asthma. Thirdly, Dr Warmhands could herself try to establish, through convergent validity, the value of peak flow as a measure of asthma. What factors should correlate? A

history of wheezing? Expiratory wheezes heard with the stethoscope?, etc.

In addition, she should consider what other diseases may produce a lowered peak-flow and should try and introduce a question or test to distinguish these diseases from asthma. This might be termed *divergent* or *discriminant* validity.

Basically, then, there can be two different ways of measuring asthma.

1.   We might have a single indicator, say peak flow, which we know from corroborative evidence identifies asthmatics. The peak-flow meter reading therefore becomes the criterion we would adopt.

2.   We may decide that asthma requires more than one indicator because either peak-flow readings miss some cases or also include other diseases. We might then say that asthma exists if the following conditions are met:

- there is a peak-flow reading below x;
- there is a history of wheezing;
- the stethoscope reveals bronchial wheezes.

(4)   Eczema

The control group of eczematous children poses similar problems of definition. What is to count as eczema and how severe does it have to be before it can be considered an appropriate control for asthma? Again, recourse to a dermatology textbook or previous research on eczema may provide useful criteria for deciding what is eczema and what is not, although there may be 'mixed' or unclear skin lesions which cannot be precisely diagnosed. In addition, there is the problem of measuring severity. Eczema may be a $1 \, cm^2$ patch on the back of a hand or it may cover a large surface of the body. If there is not a 'meter' with which to measure it, how can we decide?

First, Dr Warmhands needs to make a judgement as to whether or not eczema is present. Next, she must devise fairly precise rules for making a clinical judgement on its severity. Thus she might say that the severity of eczema should be scored on a three-point scale:

1 = mild, patient relatively unconcerned, no interference with their lives;
2 = moderate, covers some sensitive body areas, patient concerned, needs treatment;
3 = severe, widespread, incapacitating, topical steroids necessary to control.

Perhaps those scoring 2 or 3 on the scale could join the control group.

Is this measurement practical? Yes, it can be carried out easily during the consultation.

Is it reliable? Assuming the lesion remained constant over a couple of weeks, reliability of the measure could be tested by seeing if an assessment on one occasion agreed with assessment on another. In practice the disease is likely to change over time, so such checks may be difficult. How else could the consistency of this particular measure be assessed?

If Dr Warmhands were clearly to describe the scale of mild, moderate, and severe to two of her partners she could ask them to score the same patients as she does and then compare results. If the results are consistently the same then the instrument (in effect a GP applying the scale) is reliable.

She could go further and ask two local dermatologists to help with the study. Again, she would have to spend time with them agreeing what is to count as eczema and how they will work the severity scale. Then each case could be scored by five people: Dr Warmhands, her two partners, and the two dermatologists. Each would score eczema present or absent, and, if present, what degree of severity (1, 2, or 3).

In practice, this would be a rather involved procedure just to establish a control group, but the principle of using separate raters is a useful one for measuring something rather nebulous. It could be used, for example, in scoring a patient's quality of life if several raters all listen to a tape recording of a patient describing their life. There is a special term, 'inter-rater reliability', which describes the degree of agreement between different raters. These techniques will be covered in more depth in later chapters.

For the present it is sufficient to know that comparison of trained raters can be used to test reliability. Perhaps the word *trained* should be emphasized, because assessing reliability in this way does depend on all the raters working the same way and, in effect, being tantamount to the same instrument. Pause for a moment and consider what would happen if your partners and the friendly dermatologists had not been 'trained'? In such a case the different assessments of the eczema by all five observers would not give a measure of reliability but of convergent validity: if, independently, they all agree on cases of, say, severe eczema then clearly your assessments are valid.

In summary, two *similar* measurements of the same phenomenon can be used to assess reliability, two *different* measurements, convergent validity. The difficulty can arise of whether two measures are sufficiently similar to assess reliability or sufficiently dissimilar to assess validity. Is your training of your dermatology colleagues sufficient? If it is, they can help you assess reliability. If it is not, then they can help you establish validity.

(5) Parent
Parent would again be operationalized in the light of the hypothesis. In a genetic study, parent no doubt would imply biological parent; in this study Dr Warmhands presumably means whoever is responsible for 'parenting'

the child. In addition she is looking for a relationship between 'parents' so she needs two of them.

Thus she might define parents as a man and woman who have been looking after the child, as parents, during the past three years. This could be established from asking the child or the 'parents' who accompany the child. Reliability is likely to be high and face validity is probably sufficient here.

(6)   *Interpersonal relationship*
Concepts such as child, parent, attendance, etc. are relatively easy to operationalize: first they are fairly low-level concepts—they almost define themselves—so face validity is good, and secondly there is a good degree of consensus as to what the terms mean anyway. With concepts such as the quality of interpersonal relationships there are greater problems: the concept is very abstract so operationalizing can be difficult, and because the exact meaning of the term is not clear there are likely to be as many indicators as there are meanings.

How can something as abstract as interpersonal relationships be measured?

Most measurement in medicine concerns physical things, bodies, diseases, biological parameters, etc., and these can seem easier to measure than psychosocial ones because they can somehow be 'seen'. But this view is rather simplistic. Blood pressure might be biological/physical but in fact it cannot be seen. Clinicians put a device, the sphygmomanometer, between them and the blood pressure to make it visible. This is precisely the process described above whereby concepts are operationalized as indicators, so achieving practical ways in which they can be measured.

The measurement of social relationships can be approached in exactly the same way. Leaving aside for the moment the possibility of actually observing the relationship, how can Dr Warmhands transform the relationship as it exists in the parents' heads to an indicator that will express the relationship as a number, just as the sphygmomanometer translates the concept of blood pressure into so many millimetres of mercury? These principles are important because they can be used to transform any mental state—anxiety, depression, satisfaction, joy, etc.—into numbers which can then be used in research. Problems of validity are more important here but we shall approach these shortly. For the moment let us take the problem of how to convert thoughts into numbers—specifically, the views of a parent on the quality of the relationship they have with their spouse into some sort of numerical scale.

First proceed as in the physical sciences: there is a phenomenon Dr Warmhands wishes to measure, therefore she has to devise an appropriate instrument (through operationalizing the concept), and then go ahead and measure it. A very simple instrument might be the question:

Q.1. 'Do you have a good marriage?'

There are, as you might guess, some difficulties with this approach which do not occur for the natural scientist.

The problem of meaning

Measuring the length of several pencils is straightforward because the characteristic, length, is constant in each pencil and between different pencils. With human beings, however, the object under study is not a passive constant: people are constantly changing and, moreover, they evaluate stimuli before reacting to them. In other words before replying to a question, people inevitably evaluate the question ('What does it mean?') before replying. The pencil is not aware of the presence or intentions of the ruler, whereas people are aware of the presence of the researcher's instrument and infer intentions in the researcher. Thus if someone believes the mark of a good marriage is to have lots of children, their response to the question will, unknown to the researcher, be misleading.

Dr Warmhands therefore needs to develop some special techniques to try and manage this problem of meaning. It might be pointed out at this stage that some social researchers have argued that this problem is insuperable and that such research is always flawed. They would be more inclined to adopt the qualitative methods outlined in the previous and in later chapters. Our position is that while there are difficulties there are ways of at least minimizing them.

In essence, the problem of meaning potentially interferes with the validity of our chosen instrument, as Dr Warmhands may not be measuring the phenomenon she thinks she is measuring, but rather her respondents' own idiosyncratic interpretations of her instrument. She therefore has to be very careful about the process of operationalization and the checks on validity. Let us go through the process step by step.

Concept: 'quality of a relationship'
(Thinks: What does this actually mean?)
Operationalize
Indicator: 'Do you have a good marriage?)

This indicator has face validity, but it has various limitations:

- It is open to the patient's own interpretation of what is actually meant by the word 'good'.
- It is a rather narrow operationalization: as given in the initial hypothesis, the quality of a relationship implied something much wider; in fact it might be argued that we started with a multidimensional concept and produced a unidimensional indicator, a bit like measuring a box with only one of its three dimensions.

In the light of this, the question does seem inadequate. It can be improved by replacing it with a question which is more specific. In addition, given that the concept is multidimensional, she might try more than one question to tap different facets of the quality of a marriage. Try:

Q.2.   *'Do you often have rows?'*
Q.3.   *'If you have a problem, can you talk it over with your partner?'*

Together these two questions constitute a very elementary questionnaire. How has she improved on the first instrument?

- Because of patient interpretation of Question 1, it seemed likely to give an invalid result. Questions 2 and 3 are more focused and perhaps less subject to interpretation problems.
- This seems to be a better operationalization than Question 1. Already she is beginning to tap two important features of a relationship: does it suffer from breakdowns and is it generally supportive?

Of course she could go on adding questions to our questionnaire, each one tapping a different facet of what the researcher thinks might be the quality of the relationship. In principle the more questions, the better the questionnaire but, as we shall see in Chapter 4, there are some practical constraints.

For the moment Dr Warmhands decides to stop at her two-question— or, as it is often called, *item*—questionnaire. She might ask one patient's parent 'Do you often have rows?' and they might reply 'Not particularly'. Whatever does this mean? The problem of meaning can be seen to be a two-way phenomenon: the respondent must interpret the researcher's question and the researcher must in turn interpret the answer.

A series of patients might provide a series of answers to Question 1: 'Not particularly', 'Yes', 'Never, except over money', 'Less than might be expected', and so on. Dr Warmhands obviously needs to ensure that the responses she elicits make sense in terms of some sort of scale. The commonest way of achieving this is to provide a series of set answers and ask the respondent to choose the one closest to their answer. Thus she might have:

'Do you often have rows?'   Yes   ☐
                                                                  No   ☐

(Please tick the appropriate box)

The difficulty with constraining respondents in this way is that in trying to avoid ambiguous answers she has imposed her own measuring system. Perhaps the respondent has rows twice a year: is that to count as 'often'? What exactly is meant by 'rows' and by 'often'?

In effect there are two extreme ways of working: one can ask short questions which force responses into perhaps inappropriate categories, or invite the respondent simply to talk about their rows, record these on tape and count this as the data collection. Thus:

- 'Do you often have rows?'   Yes/No
- 'Tell me about any rows you have?'   (tape on)

These two approaches can be differentiated as *structured* and *unstructured*. The latter will require considerable analysis and 'structuring' *after* data collection—a topic to be covered in Chapter 6. For the moment let us stay with Dr Warmhand's structured questionnaire.

It is clear that the structured questionnaire and response frame she has devised above is very short and crude. How can it be improved?

She could of course add new questions to tap other aspects of the relationship, or indeed, further questions to clarify the questions already asked, such as exactly what is meant by rows. Perhaps:

'Do you ever quarrel about money?'
'Do you have disagreements about child care?'
'Do you believe occasional arguments help to clear the air?
And so on.

In addition, she can widen the response frame to include a wider choice: she could provide five boxes to tick rather than two, etc. Specific details of questionnaire design will be covered in Chapter 4.

CONSTRUCT VALIDITY

It is clear that there is considerable potential latitude in the design of a questionnaire to measure something such as the quality of a relationship. The actual type and numbers of individual items can vary considerably. How do the researchers know when they have got it right? How do we know when we are actually measuring the things we set out to measure, in this case the quality of a relationship?

The problem is that if we fail to show any connection between asthma and parental relationships it could be:

(1) because there isn't one;

(2) because we failed to measure the quality of relationships (or asthma) adequately.

It is impossible to know which of the two is the answer. However, if on the other hand we find that there *is* a connection between asthma and quality of relationships, then we have, in effect, shown that our operationalization worked and was in some sense valid. Of course, it may not have measured precisely what we thought it had measured, but having shown a connection we are obviously onto something which we can pursue.

Let us take this argument through its steps again. Say we have a hypothesis that: 'Wimps are only found among men.'

1.   We need a research design and a sample. Let us take the next consecutive 100 men and 100 women who consult, check who is a wimp and compare the two groups.

2.   We need to operationalize our variables—namely, men, women, and wimpishness. Men and women we shall identify from our case records; only people over 18 will be eligible. When our grandmothers were not sucking eggs they did offer the insight that cats do not like wimps: we shall therefore observe the behaviour of a cat when these 200 people enter the consulting room.

3.   We collect our data. Pickles, the surgery cat, ran out of the room when seven out of the 100 men entered and when two of the 100 women entered.

4.   Thus, looked at formally, either our initial hypothesis has been disproved (because we hypothesized that wimps were never found amongst women) or the cat has not proved to be a very valid instrument. Which is it? Let's try a new cat.

5.   We hire a new cat and repeat the experiment. This cat runs out of the room when six of the men enter but never when a woman enters. Our hypothesis is confirmed. And we can be more sure the new cat can somehow identify wimps better than the old one. (The cat may, in fact, be detecting the presence of aftershave for all we know—we do know, however, that whatever it does, it does better than the old cat.)

Now apply the same logic to Dr Warmhands's relationship questionnaire. Assume that she uses her two-item questionnaire to assess quality of relationships. If she has allowed a two-point response frame and scores these 0 or 1, then adding the two items together she gets a scale of 0–2 for quality of marriage. Let us assume the overall results are as follows:

20 asthmatic children:	average marriage score = 1.3
20 eczematous children:	average marriage score = 1.4

The quality of relationships in her control group is slightly better but hardly very much. She would be safe in saying there was no difference. What does this imply? Either:

- her hypothesis is mistaken; or
- her relationship instrument was too crude to pick up the subtleties she was after

Now consider some other results:

20 asthmatic children:	average marriage score = 0.3
20 eczematous children:	average marriage score = 1.8

The results, and hence implications, are very different. She might still rightly be sceptical of her 'relationship' instrument but it has certainly picked something up. Now she can ask 'What is it?' What is it about a relationship which has been identified? Is it something to do with rows specifically? Is it something to do with communication? Once more she must return to her hypothesis because suddenly it looks far too general, and in the light of how the quality of relationships was operationalized she must try new hypotheses and new instruments to refine what she has identified.

On these grounds a questionnaire is sufficient if it can help to identify links between variables at both an empirical and theoretical level. The thought behind the hypothesis was that perhaps a poor marital background actually caused or exacerbated asthma. Thus:

$$\text{poor parental interaction} \longrightarrow \text{asthma}$$

These concepts were operationalized and measured. Thus:

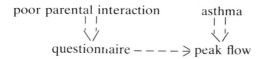

A relationship was then found between the questionnaire findings and the peak-flow reading. Assuming this has not occurred by chance—and this is established by statistical techniques explored in Chapter 8—we have stumbled across something quite interesting because the link between the very specific measures indicates a link between the more fuzzy concepts. This phenomenon is called *construct validity* because it is known from the correlation between the measures that the hypothesis or construct has some validity.

The above examples are rather simple because they are based only on a two-variable relationship (i.e. parental relationships and asthma). In practice, construct validity is usually explored in the context of several supposedly related variables. Thus, for instance, it can be seen from the above example that, if there is a positive correlation between the relationship questionnaire and asthma, there is some support for the value of the relationship concept and how it was operationalized. But if, in addition, the questionnaire is used to identify couples with and without marital problems and then compares these for depression, and again a correlation is found, there is even more support for the concept and its operationalization. Clearly this process can go on and on, each new variable which can be linked to our concept reinforcing its validity, and gradually establishing a matrix of corroborative support for all the variables.

Construct validity is therefore important in two ways:

- when dealing with rather woolly concepts it offers some supportive evidence that the operationalization is adequate;
- because research is ultimately about building hypotheses into wider explanatory models, construct validity provides the bridge between measuring things and developing wider theories (often containing many variables) about the world.

If a positive correlation between two variables is found, it is not the end of the research process but a sort of beginning. What has really been shown? What concept did the indicator really measure? Like bloodhounds following a scent the researcher has to decide constantly in which direction to go. If a trail has no scent, should it be abandoned or examined even more closely for a scent that may have been missed? If, on the other hand, a scent is discovered, its direction must be determined and then pursued.

Usually, in research data are collected on more than two variables so that if a trail is found it can be explored further without going immediately back into the field. Thus if there does seem to be a correlation between parental relationships and asthma, the data can be used to ask additional questions:

'Does it hold for boys and girls?'
'Is it age related?'
And so on.

In this sense research is never completed: it goes on, one question leading to another, one finding suggesting another or a new line of enquiry.

SUMMARY

This chapter has dealt with the process by which the abstract terms or concepts in a research design are transposed into practical measuring procedures. These stages are:

(1)   operationalizing individual concepts to create measurable indicators;
(2)   paying attention to the validity of this operationalization by checking wherever possible by:
- face validity;
- convergent validity.
(3)   We see if we have a positive correlation between elements in our hypothesis.

If there is not a correlation:
- we discuss or change our hypothesis;

- we rethink our operationalization;
- we add in some more checks for validity.

If there is a correlation:

- we have some construct validity;
- we proceed to refine our hypothesis;
- we refine and further develop our operationalization;
- we use our new measures to collect data;
- we check for new correlations.

SUGGESTED TASKS

1.   Design and carry out a study to assess the reliability of sphygmoma-nometers both in the surgery and in doctors' bags. You might also try interperson variability in the reading of a blood pressure.

2.   For the next 10 investigations you order, try and predict the result. See if your clinical impression is as valid as the test.

ANSWERS TO EXERCISES

Exercise 3(1)

Concept	*Indicator*
income	monthly net salary
elderly	aged over 65
women	presence of a vagina
	reported gender
stress	galvanic skin resistance
	heart rate
chronic illness	on disability register
	reports long-standing illness
GP workload	length of surgeries
	number of patients seen
referral rate	patients sent to OP
blood pressure	sphygmomanometer reading

Exercise 3(2)

1.   Aged over 65; any glycosuria?
2.   (Difficult ... what do we mean by concentration?) Each patient is given a short message by receptionist to give to the doctor. Doctor recalls the message at the end of the consultation. Compare recall in the first half hour of surgery with that of the last half hour.

3. Compare the numbers of each patients aged over 65 in your age–sex registers.

4. Identify high- and low-stressed patients by a stress questionnaire: compare the consultation rates from notes made over the last year. (Remember to balance your groups—high consulters are more likely to enter your sample if you use surgery patients.)

5. Divide hand movement in 'types': e.g. over chest, flat; over chest, fisted; not over chest.

   For patients presenting with chest pain record type of hand movement, then make diagnosis, e.g. with ECG; does a particular hand movement correlate with ECG ischaemic changes? (If it does then there is some construct validity to the concept of 'diagnostic hand movements' which might be worth exploring further.)

Exercise 3(3)

Q.1. Face validity.

Q.2. Convergent (concurrent) validity.

Q.3. Convergent (predictive) validity.

Q.4. Convergent (concurrent) validity.

Q.5. Face validity.

4 Collecting data

The previous chapter dealt with deciding how you might go about measuring things. Having made those decisions you are almost ready to go 'into the field' to measure things in practice. But before you do so you have to give some thought to how you are going to collect your data. 'Data' are 'out there'. You will need some sort of 'net' to bring data in: the net must be the right size and its mesh dimensions appropriate for the data you want to capture. This chapter deals with designing this 'net' for collecting data.

COLLECTING AND CLASSIFYING DATA

It is reported that if a blind person is given his or her sight back, initially they can see only a blur. Gradually they begin to recognize objects and eventually they can 'see'.

Sensory data surround us in an undiscriminated mass. As our perceptual processes develop—usually in childhood—we begin to organize this blur of information and we are able to identify separate objects, colours, textures, sounds, etc. In effect, being able to see is not simply allowing images to flood our retinas—that would produce a haze—but using our brain to organize and select elements of visual data so that we can identify a recognizable picture. Of course there must be a sensory input through the retina but the image is 'manufactured' in the visual cortex.

Research is exactly analogous. Out there are data, masses and masses of the stuff. And one of the commonest mistakes of those not versed in research methods is to imagine that research is about having a data receptor—like a retina—which will enable giant spoonfuls of data to be captured.

'I've collected serum rhubarb estimations on over 600 patients.' 'Have you? I've done it on over 800!' 'Wow!' What a big research grant/team/programme you must have!'

But so what? Chapter 1 stressed that you must start your research with a question. This is the point when perseverance pays off. Certainly you need to collect data, but the research question (together with the research design, Chapter 2, and how the concepts were operationalized, Chapter 3) will help you to decide which data you are going to collect and how you are going to organize a picture from it all.

Data collection always involves some selectivity or organization; collecting 'random' data is feasible but clearly absurd. Nevertheless it is useful to distinguish between the collection of data and their categorization. By and large it would seem reasonable to ensure that data were categorized before organizing their collection, so as to obtain only the exact data that are needed. However, in general-practice research, especially when collecting data from people, there may be good grounds for collecting rather un-differentiated data, and sorting and categorizing later, away from the heat of the moment.

Let us consider two examples of measuring how satisfied patients are with their last consultation in general practice.

1.   Tape record a one-hour interview with a patient in which you ask them to talk about their last consultation, its good points and bad points, and about their views of general practice in general. Let the patient do most of the talking: only prompt with open-ended questions or facilitating statements.

2.   Give a patient a questionnaire to complete. The questionnaire contains the question:

'Were you satisfied with your last consultation?'   Yes ☐

No ☐

(Please tick the appropriate box)

With both of these approaches the data are 'out there' mixed in with all sorts of other data, such as opinions on baked beans, politicians, and shrubs. The research question boils down to abstracting from this amorphous mass whether or not the patient was satisfied with the last consultation.

In the first example (1) the data collected on an hour-long tape record-ing were sufficiently focused so as to be mainly about general practice, but beyond that not sufficiently categorized to answer the research question ('Was the patient satisfied?') without further work by the researcher to disentangle relevant data from background 'noise'. In example 2, on the other hand, the data were collected and categorized at exactly the same time. Indeed, by giving the patient a self-administered questionnaire we succeeded in getting the patient to organize the data for us.

The popularity of questionnaires that are self-administered and 'struc-tured' (in that they require the patient simply to answer closed questions) is no doubt due primarily to the ease by which data collection and organiza-tion are achieved in one simple exercise (using the respondent as a sort of unpaid research assistant). However, this sort of data collection/ organization has limitations, and in many ways example 1 may give a 'better' result. Example 2 depends on the patient as untrained researcher to do the classification for us. But is this wise? Patients may misinterpret the question, they might think we are trying to find out whether they got well or were given a prescription, and answer accordingly. Example 1 allows *us* to do the classifying according to consistent and more rigorous criteria. Moreover, potentially it allows us to ask more interesting questions, such as 'What was it exactly that the patient found satisfying?'

The choice is therefore between relatively complex data-collection methods, which may produce good quality data but where complexity means we may have to restrict sample size, and more simple techniques, which allow large numbers of cases to make up for any insensitivity in the measuring instrument. Whichever method is used will be strongly influenced by the precise nature of the research question being asked. Without doubt, collecting data on patients' ages is best done using a question which asks the patient to give an answer properly categorized into the exact number of years; on the other hand, the validity of a response to the question 'What is the quality of your life?' which involved ticking one of two boxes is likely to be limited: these latter sorts of data are better collected in a more undifferentiated form.

In this chapter we are primarily concerned with data collection but inevitably some methods of collection involve quite elaborate classification as explained above, whereas others tend to deal with fairly raw material. The subsequent steps of completing categorization and carrying out further manipulation will be pursued in Chapter 6.

TYPES OF DATA COLLECTION

A new weight-reducing drug called 'Skinnyfax' has been brought onto the market recently. Results from trials indicate that it might be beneficial, although it is still unclear how it works. Does it actually cause weight reduction in everyone? Does it produce weight reduction by appetite suppression or by increasing basic metabolic rate? And what are its side-effects? There have been some reports of raised blood pressure. Dr Adrian Slim decides to set up a small research study evaluating its impact in the context of general practice.

His sample consists of those patients who consult with him and whose weights are above the 90th percentile for their age. The design involves the patients being randomized between an experimental group which receives the drug, and a group which acts as a control. (The patients will be asked if they agree to this procedure.) Part of the study will involve collecting baseline information on a range of topics so as to identify the level and nature of change (if any) produced by the drug. Dr Slim will need to collect information on patients' eating habits, weight, blood pressure, side-effects, etc., and record any changes in the experimental and control groups.

What ways are there for collecting the necessary data? Figure 4.1 shows the possibilities. Each method involves collecting data at different levels of prior categorization: data collected by relatively unstructured means will require later structuring, whereas data collected by structured means will be virtually ready for analysis.

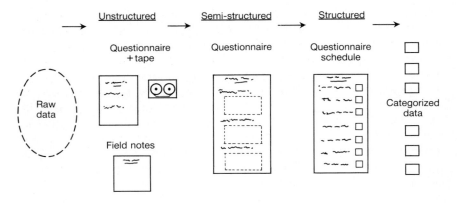

Fig. 4.1. Data collection methods.

Let us see how these different methods might work for the data needed to be collected for the Skinnyfax study, especially the data on eating habits.

Unstructured techniques

These divide into observation and interview.

Observation

When social anthropologists wish to study a community they often use techniques of 'unstructured' observation. They do not want to intrude into what is going on, for example by asking questions, because these might cause someone to change their behaviour; the preferred technique is therefore observation. Secondly, they want their observations to be unstructured because if they were to structure their collection of data, using a classification system devised before they arrived in the community, they might miss something important. Thus they start with a blank piece of paper entitled 'field notes' and write down the things they see. Of course, to stay within the bounds of the possible, some structuring is necessary, and so the researchers will only write down what they believe might be significant in the context of their purposes in hand. Arguably, this low-level selection of what to record is better and more sensitive than having a list of pre-set questions to be answered.

Similarly, in order to find out what people eat there are clear advantages to making an actual observation of what they do eat. In principle then, Dr Slim could visit their homes and, without preconceptions of what he might find, observe their behaviour. In fact this would no doubt be impracticable, but the basis of this sort of data collection, if it were feasible, is worth spelling out. (While this procedure may be unsuitable for this particular study topic it may be useful elsewhere—such as in the consulting room.)

If Dr Slim were accepted as a 'fly on the wall', he would presumably get a better idea of eating habits—perhaps the husband/father gets twice as much as anyone else—whereas a questionnaire may simply elicit some general gloss such as 'we all eat the same'. Equally, going in without preconceptions will enable surprising or unexpected events to be recorded.

After he has made his observations there are three things he can do with them:

- use these accounts in their own right, as descriptive studies that offer insights into the phenomena under study, and write them up as such (i.e. as purely qualitative studies);
- read them through carefully and use the insights they afford as the basis for a more traditional structured questionnaire to be used on a larger sample;
- analyse the field notes and transpose 'qualitative' data into quantitative by techniques described in Chapter 6.

Interview

What happens if the phenomena Dr Slim wished to explore were not behaviours but mental processes, such as attitudes, beliefs, values, etc? The method of data collection chosen is exactly analogous to unstructured observation, only this time, instead of using field notes to record data, he would use a tape recorder. With observational techniques he could observe a meal; with interview techniques, however, he obviously cannot rely on the patient suddenly talking about their attitude to food when the tape recorder is placed in front of them. Instead he would have to create the necessary conditions which encourage and enable them to talk about eating: this is done by a series of open-ended questions, prompts, facilitating reponses, etc., which written down beforehand would constitute an *unstructured questionnaire*. It might look something like this:

Eating habits questionnaire
Respondent's name:
Date:
Time:
Tape Number:

Tell me about your food shopping?
Who does it? Always? Where? How often?
Do you decide in advance what to buy?

What sorts of things do you buy?
Always? For special occasions?   etc.

Dr Slim may not, of course, need to use many of these questions should a respondent cover them spontaneously for him. Or, if the respondent starts to talk about the role of money in determining shopping patterns, it might be inappropriate to return to the planned topics, so instead the new lead would be pursued. In effect the questionnaire is just a series of prompts to ensure that the interview does not dry up, otherwise it is allowed to take its own course.

Again the results of the interview on the tape can be used as the basis of a descriptive account, transformed into quantitative data, or used to create a structured questionnaire.

Semi-structured techniques

These, as their name implies, fall midway between unstructured and structured techniques. The most important is the *semi-structured questionnaire* in which the questions are fairly well structured but unstructured responses are allowed. In other words, all respondents will get the same questions, but, as they will be open-ended, everyone will provide answers different in both content and form. Thus the question, 'Where do you do your shopping?', might elicit the response: 'Sainsburys' from one person but a five-minute monologue on grocery retailing from another. The results of semi-structured questionnaires can be analysed in the same way as unstructured techniques.

Structured techniques

Structured techniques collect data which is pre-categorized, with perhaps the best known being the structured questionnaire, but, as we shall see, many forms of data collection fall into this mode. Indeed, any piece of paper on which is written pre-categorized data is a structured technique. These are known as *schedules*.

Let us consider different forms of schedule.

A clinical schedule

The Skinnyfax study requires Dr Slim to collect some clinical data. This might include information on the patient's weight, height, blood pressure, and perhaps some laboratory investigations. He decides to collect most of these during the consultation. To record the data he collects he will therefore need to design a schedule. How might this look?

It would probably be on a single sheet of paper. It would require a title (to distinguish it from other schedules lying around the surgery?). The first entry would probably be the patient's name together with a code number which the researcher would devise. The value of having a code number as an identifier should become clearer later. (Briefly, the data is more than likely to be computerized and computers are not very good at handling people's names; instead a three-digit number would easily enable the identification of up to 999 individual patients.) Dr Slim might want the date on which he did the examination, and of course places to record the clinical data. The finished product might look something like this:

Skinnyfax study: baseline clinical data

Patient's name: Code Number:

Date:

Height (metres):
Weight (kg):

Blood pressure:
Haemoglobin:
Serum cholesterol:

(Presumably laboratory findings can be added later when the results are returned.)

The advantage of having such a schedule is that nothing is forgotten in the data collection and data is not spread over odd bits and pieces of paper. In addition, if the schedule is carefully designed, the data in the boxes can be used directly to create a data-file on a computer: the value of this will become apparent in a later chapter when we discuss how to 'code' a questionnaire.

The clinical schedule can be expanded to include data collected in the evaluation phase. Indeed, the schedule could be so designed to bring all the data on each case together on the same record.

An extraction schedule

It may be possible to obtain study data from other written sources, especially case notes. Again the source is likely to include far too much data so some sort of schedule must be designed—in this case what we might call an extraction schedule—so as to obtain precisely the data we are interested in. Its form is likely to be the same as the clinical schedule, outlined above. Indeed, if the case notes were to contain the relevant data, exactly the same schedule could be used.

Case notes are the most likely source of written data. However, case notes are primarily used for clinical and administrative purposes and thus the information recorded will be structured by these aims. There is unlikely to be, for example, the breadth of information available for a research investigation on eating habits unless some careful attempt has been made to record such data in the past. The case notes, however, could be used in this study for validity checks for weight and for other clinical information, such as blood pressure.

A structured questionnaire

Often the data to be collected has to be obtained not from patients' bodies nor from written records but from what exists in the patient's mind (attitudes, moods, values, beliefs, etc.). The common technique for doing this is the structured or standardized questionnaire, where the range of questions is structured, meaning that choice of answers is restricted. This approach stands in contrast to the unstructured interview, where there is no set order, no schedule, and the researcher is not necessarily looking for exactly the same information from each respondent.

Questionnaires are exactly analogous to any other schedule but, because it is people who are being interrogated, they must be more carefully set out and worded. Thus the question 'Height: ...' which was sufficient on the clinical schedule would have to be reworded: perhaps, 'What is your height in metres?' In addition, care must be taken in the design of the questionnaire to ensure maximum response rates. The sphygmomanometer is not usually in the habit of saying 'I don't think I want to measure this particular blood pressure', whereas people do have an unfortunate disposition to say 'no' to the best-intentioned research studies.

The use of a standardized questionnaire is most appropriate for collecting information:

- from a large number of people;
- from a relatively homogeneous group of people who tend to share the same general perspective and characteristics;
- in situations where you already know enough about the subject and the kinds of respondents so that you know what to ask and how to ask it.

The major limitation of this approach is when it is used with groups of respondents who do not necessarily share your values and views, and thus the assumptions which are incorporated into the questionnaire are invalid. For example, if you are looking at patterns of eating habits and the factors that influence them, you might assume that people's concern about matters of health are of paramount importance. However, this might be an invalid assumption and only reflect your concerns as a professional rather than the values and priorities of your respondents.

The questions in the structured schedule can be given to the respondents in at least two ways. The questionnaire can be given directly to the respondents for them to complete themselves (*a self-administered questionnaire*) or it can be given by a trained intermediary (*an interviewer-administered questionnaire*). Self-administered questionnaires are particularly useful for collecting relatively straightforward information from a large sample, quickly and cheaply. On the other hand, an interviewer-administered questionnaire tends to produce a higher response rate (80 per cent on average) and better-quality information. Also the questionnaire itself could be more complicated as the interviewer would be on hand to explain the questions. However, it is more time-consuming and expensive, not least because you have to recruit, pay, and train the interviewers.

Question 4(1)

Dr Slim feels that his survey on eating habits should be simple and he is confident that the use of a standardized questionnaire is appropriate. However, he has to decide on how to gather the information. Should he use:

(a) a self-administered postal questionnaire; or
(b) an interviewer-administered questionnaire?

Self-administered questionnaires can be handed out in person, e.g. in the surgery, but this restricts the sample to patients who consult; alternatively, they can be sent by post. Certainly, a postal questionnaire has some advantages over interviews.

1. Postal questionnaires are generally cheaper and quicker.
2. Postal questionnaires are useful with large and widely distributed sample, e.g. a national sample.

However, there are also some disadvantages with a postal questionnaire.

1. The response is rarely as high as in interview studies, as there is less incentive to respond. The average response rate in a postal questionnaire is around 50–60 per cent.
2. The quality of response to the questionnaire may be variable and there is no guarantee that the selected individual will be the member of the household who has filled it in.

If a postal questionnaire is used, emphasis would be placed on trying to maximise the response rate. Much will depend on the covering letter that is sent with the questionnaire and, in addition, follow-up reminders will need to be sent out.

For example, here is a letter which might be sent with a postal questionnaire on health habits:

Dear Sir or Madam,

We are writing to ask for your help with a health survey which the Rundown Health Authority is carrying out with Smallbrick University.

It is the responsibility of the Health Authority to promote health and prevent disease as well as to treat illness when it occurs, and it makes good sense to do so. We want to find out more about the general health of our community and about factors which may affect people's health, such as smoking, diet, exercise, and drinking. By filling in this questionnaire about your health you will help us to do this and, in due course, to improve the health of the community.

We obviously cannot send out questionnaires to every person living in Rundown so we have carefully taken a random sample which should be representative of the District as a whole. It is important to us that you fill in your questionnaire and return it as your replies are essential in building up the overall picture.

You will find that most questions are simple to answer, requiring just a tick in a box, although any extra comments you may wish to make will be welcome.

Your reply will be handled in strict confidence. This means that your name will not appear on the questionnaire, it will be handled only by authorized members of the research staff and your answers will not be seen by your GP or any other person. The questionnaire will be shredded after use and no individuals will be identified or identifiable in any reports or publications. When you have returned the questionnaire there will be no further communication from us.

The replies will be analysed in the Health Services Research Unit of Smallbrick University and we will be grateful if you return your completed questionnaire in the enclosed envelope.

May we thank you in advance for the time and trouble taken in completing this questionnaire.

Yours faithfully,

The letter tells the respondent:

(1) who is carrying out the survey;
(2) why the survey is being carried out and its value;
(3) why the individual has been selected;
(4) how to fill in the questionnaire;
(5) about confidentiality and anonymity;
(6) where to return the questionnaire.

On most occasions one attempted contact with the respondent is not sufficient to obtain a good-enough response rate in a postal survey. The first follow-up, usually a short letter or a postcard, is sent 2–3 weeks after the letter and questionnaire are sent. The main aim is to jog the memory of those who intended to complete the questionnaire but have either forgotten or have not found the time.

The second follow-up usually involves a more persuasive covering letter with another copy of the questionnaire. It, too, has the aim of reminding respondents, although it is also aimed at the hard core of non-respondents, attempting to persuade them to take part. Using more than two follow-ups is not usually cost-effective, in that the time and money spent on sending out letters and paying for return envelopes does not normally justify the small increase in the response rate.

In general, the following factors are believed to increase response rates (and conversely their absence decrease it):

- the more independent and prestigious the sponsoring body (universities tend to do better than commercial market research organizations);
- the brevity of the questionnaire (shorter the better);
- identification of the respondent with the area of the research (a questionnaire on skin diseases will elicit a better response from those concerned about their skin than those not);
- ease of completion (clear instructions, easy and rapid marking, a stamped-addressed return envelope, etc.);
- payment or financial incentive (though these are rarely paid).

After weighing up his choices Dr Slim decides to use a postal questionnaire to assess his patients' eating habits.

HOW DO YOU CONSTRUCT A QUESTIONNAIRE?

Designing a self-administered questionnaire can be a slow process when you do not have the skills of the interviewer to mediate between the questionnaire and the respondent. How do you go about it?

A title

The questionnaire should have a title both to identify it for your benefit, but also so that the respondent will have some idea of what it is about. Keep it short and clear: 'Satisfaction survey', 'Self-medication questionnaire', etc. Dr Slim chooses 'Eating habits questionnaire'.

An address

If you are carrying out a postal survey, you should provide an address somewhere in the questionnaire, often just under the title. Do not rely on the address on a covering letter as these get mislaid. Even for questionnaires handed out in the surgery it is useful to have a name and/or address in case the patient inadvertently walks out without handing it in. Dr Slim puts, under his title:

> please return to:
> Dr Adrian Slim
> Puddleton Health Centre

An identifier

There should be a box somewhere near the beginning of the questionnaire in which can be written the respondent's code number. This is used as an identifier so that one respondent's questionnaire can easily be distinguished from any other. This is particularly useful in postal surveys for sending out reminder letters or postcards (to those numbers not replying to a first mailing), or in constructing the data-file (see Chapter 6). Dr Slim's survey is of 500 patients so he places a box to take a three-digit number in the top right-hand corner of the questionnaire, where it is easily visible.

Some instructions

The first section of any questionnaire should also tell respondents something about the survey and how to complete the questionnaire. This should be as clear and as simple as possible. Dr Slim prefaces the questions with the following remarks:

We are carrying out a survey of people's eating habits in this practice and we would be grateful for your help. Can you please answer the following questions. Most simply require a tick in the appropriate boxes.

All your answers will be treated in the strictest confidence. Thank you for helping.

Alternatively, in a postal questionnaire some of these details could be described in the covering letter.

The questions

The next stage involves constructing the actual questions. This requires the identification of the particular topics needed for the questionnaire, and then these need formalizing into specific questions.

(1) *What topics do I wish to cover in the questionnaire?* Dr Slim has decided that in his study of patients' eating habits he wants to divide the topic area of study into the food that they buy, the way food is prepared for meals, and the type of meals that are eaten. He is also interested in social and demographic characteristics of his patients and how they vary with eating habits; so he adds social class, income, age, sex, household size, and marital status to his checklist.

(2) *What specific questions should I ask and how should they be worded?* The specific questions asked will be related to the topics and items listed previously. There are some general rules for asking questions:

- Keep the questions as short and as specific as possible.
- Use simple language.
- Avoid leading questions.
- Avoid inviting a single response to what are in fact two questions: e.g. 'Do you like meat and vegetables?'

Many questions are straightforward, especially ones which elicit simple facts. For example, 'How old are you?' is clear and unambiguous. If the questionnaire consists of these types of questions, then it is only necessary to make sure that the wording is clear, the question is answerable, an appropriate place or box is indicated for the response, and all questions are neatly laid out.

Question 4(2)

Which of the following questions could be used in your survey?

1. Do you have milk delivered or do you drive to the supermarket?
2. Is the meat/fish you buy usually: fresh salmon, caviar, veal, or pheasant?

3. Please list all the restaurant/cafes you have eaten in, what you ate, who you were with and how much you spent?
4. Should working people have a regular, balanced diet?
5. What are your shops like?
6. Do you prefer high levels of saturated or polyunsaturated fatty acids in your diet?
7. Why do you think being overweight is unhealthy?
8. You don't think doctors should give more advice on smoking do you?

The answer is none, as there are problems with all of them.

(a) is a double question which contains two different parts;
(b) offers a restricted and limited choice which may be irrelevant to the group you are investigating;
(c) contains too many different questions and they need to be separated;
(d) contains too many words where the meaning of the words is unclear, such as 'working', 'regular', and 'balance';
(e) is too broad and needs to be more specific;
(f) has too much jargon;
(g) is a leading question;
(h) your preferences and biases influence the answer.

Often, however, questions seek opinions and these tend to require a little more thought. A knowledge of the different types of questions and some possible formats can help in designing these sorts of questions.

Questions divide into two broad types, *closed* and *open*. The former, fixed choice, or what are sometimes called *pre-coded*, questions require the respondent to place his or her answer within a given range of choices. The latter are 'open' to any answer the respondent wishes to give.

Closed questions

To a certain extent the exact choice of question format will depend on the nature of the study in hand, although much of the choice is fairly arbitrary. Try different sorts. Here are some formats you might want to consider:

Q.1. Do you think that your diet can influence your health?
(Please tick)

Yes ☐
No ☐

The yes/no response is perhaps the most basic question format that can be used. As long as the subject is appropriate it is fairly easy and quick to answer. The only problem comes—as in all closed questions—when there is not a response category to fit the respondent's view. A not uncommon reaction when answering yes/no questions is to feel unsure (Can diet really influence health?). With only two choices the uncertain respondent is either forced into ticking the box which is nearest their view, or of ignoring the question. Therefore, the choice for the researcher is between forcing a decision (perhaps with a statement in the introduction requesting respondents to tick the box which is nearest to their view), or providing a third box for the undecided. Thus:

Q.2.   Do you think your diet can influence your health?
       (Please tick)

                                                    Yes   ☐
                                                    No   ☐
                                            Uncertain   ☐

A problem with the above question is that there is no way of differentiating between those who think diet is very influential and those you think it has a minor role, as both will have ticked 'Yes'. A common way round this is to offer a *scale*: perhaps, 'Yes, a lot' and 'Yes, a little'. Here is another example:

Q.3.   Are you eating a different diet from last year?
       (Please circle answer)
       Definitely   1
       Small change only   2
       No change   3
       Not sure   4

Here the respondent is offered a scale consisting of three numbers to record the extent of the change (plus a number for the unsure). This question could just as easily have been answered by ticking boxes; the advantage of using numbers is that these digits can be transferred directly to the data-file when the questionnaires are being processed (see Chapter 6). The disadvantage with numbers is that it might appear confusing to the respondent that 'unsure' (a 4) is somehow 'more' than 'no change' (a 3).

Another common question format is that based around a Likert scale:

Q.4.   To what extent do you agree with the following statement:
       'Fat people tend to be happier than thin people.'
       Strongly agree   1
       Agree   2
       Uncertain   3
       Disagree   4
       Strongly disagree   5

Usually the scale consists of a number of statements (or items) which are both positive (in this case favouring obesity) and negative. Scores are allocated to each response on each item and, so long as each question referred to the same phenomenon, e.g. obesity, the scores can be summed (after allowing for whether the question was in negative or positive format).

Another variant of a self-administered scale is the *visual analogue scale* where respondents are asked to mark a point (by a cross or a circle) on a scale to indicate their answer.

Q.5.   Do you think that obesity is important in causing ill-health? Please mark a point on the line below.

Unimportant   Very important

```
 ├──────┼──────┼──────┼──────┼──────┼──────┤
 1      2      3      4      5      6      7
```

Another type of graphic rating scale is the semantic differential. This is another way of identifying repondents' attitudes to particular concepts. For example, if the concept being explored was obesity, the scale might look like this:

Q.6.   How do you think of obese people? Look at the pair of words given below and mark on the line, between each pair, the point that represents your view.

e.g. If you have to consider whether obese people tend to be funny or serious, and your view is that they are somewhere in the middle but perhaps a bit on the serious side you might answer as below:

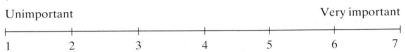

Funny   ├────┼────┼────┼────┤   Serious

Now please do the same for the following pairs of adjectives.

Good	├────┼────┼────┼────┤	Bad
Attractive	├────┼────┼────┼────┤	Ugly
Healthy	├────┼────┼────┼────┤	Unhealthy
Happy	├────┼────┼────┼────┤	Unhappy
Relaxed	├────┼────┼────┼────┤	Anxious

The example shows that the semantic differential consists of pairs of adjectives which are opposites. Each respondent is asked to mark on the five-point scales their rating of obesity in relation to the adjectives involved. The position can then be given scores of 1 to 5. Each scale can be treated independently, or the scales are often combined to see if a more general factor can be identified.

Another strategy is to ask respondents to grade or order items:

Q.7.   Which of the following vegetables do you prefer to eat?
(Please rank in order of preference)

Potatoes   Carrots   Peas   Beans   Cabbage

1st choice ....

2nd choice ....

3rd choice ....

Yet another type of question involves dividing the respondents into groups and directing one group to another question:

Q.8.   Do you eat meat?   Yes   ☐
                                                                     No   ☐

If 'yes', do you eat meat every day?	Yes ☐
	No ☐
If 'no', have you ever eaten meat?	Yes ☐
	No, never ☐

This is an example of a filter question, where the respondents are divided into subgroups and asked different clusters of questions. The question could then divide into other subgroups such as by type of meat eaten, although it is better in a self-administered questionnaire to ensure that the questioning is not too complicated.

Questions may also be included in the questionnaire to check the consistency or *internal reliability* of the questionnaire. For example, this question:

Q.9. Government regulation of additives in food is desirable.
(Please circle answer)
Agree   1
Disagree   2
Don't know   3

might be followed later by:

Q.10. Additives in food should not be regulated by the government.
(Please circle answer)
Agree   1
Disagree   2
Don't know   3

Such questions act as checks on the performance of the respondent. If the above questions elicited contradictory responses, it might suggest that the respondent is guessing (perhaps because the question is not understood) or is not taking the exercise seriously. Either of these would be a signal to treat the respondent as a 'non-responder'.

Open questions
Open questions do not constrain the respondent to answer according to the limited response set of the closed question.

Q.10 Do you think that the diet you eat can influence your health?
....
....

This is the same question as Q.1, above, but because a fixed choice response is not provided the respondent is invited to answer in any way he or she likes. The main advantage of such open-ended questions is that they do not make prior judgements about the way the respondent should answer. The main disadvantage is that they are difficult and time-consuming to code and analyse (see Chapter 6). In many ways they are probably better suited to an interview survey rather than to a self-administered questionnaire, in that the interviewer will have the opportunity of further exploring partial or unclear answers.

The ending

Sometimes, especially with lots of closed questions, respondents can get angry or frustrated that the available questions or limited choice of responses does not cover their particular interest or view. It is therefore often useful to offer a very open question right at the end:

'Do you have any further points to make about this questionnaire?'

....

Many respondents will ignore this question, others will let off steam, and yet others will offer insightful comments on the subject of the research or the details of the questionnaire. Thus while the responses are often of limited value insofar as the specifics of the questionnaire are concerned, they can be therapeutic for both respondent and researcher.

Respondents fill in questionnaires usually for no personal benefit: they are doing the researcher a favour and it is appropriate to thank them at the end.

'Thank you for helping with this study.'

The layout

Having designed all the components of the questionnaire, the next stage is to put them all together. Of course, it is almost hardly worth saying, the questionnaire should appear neat, clear and attractive. There is often a compromise to be made between spacing it out well and not letting it appear too long. In addition, some of the items will need to be ordered.

Question 4(3)

In what order do you place the following questions?
(a)   What is your income?
(b)   Where do you buy your shopping?   local shops
                                                                         supermarket
(c)   What are the best ways of staying healthy?
(d)   How do you get to the shops?   car
                                                                                bus
                                                                              other

The usual order is to place the more impersonal and easy to answer questions at the start, to enlist co-operation and gain interest, i.e. (b). This is usually followed by questions such as (d) which are less interesting. The 'sensitive' (a) and open-ended (c) are usually left to the end of the study. There is also a need to see the questionnaire as a whole, so linking phrases are necessary to ensure a smooth link-up between sections. For example, the interviewer or the text might say 'The previous question asked about the food you buy, the next group of questions looks at how you prepare it.'

Testing

The final stage of any questionnaire design is to test it for problems. It is vital that the whole research procedure is critically reviewed in the form of a *pilot* study, and this is covered in the next chapter. But even before this it is important to examine critically the questionnaire that has been designed. The most experienced researcher is still fully able to put silly or unanswerable questions into a questionnaire and these can only be picked up by asking other people to check it over.

Ask your spouse, your partners, your receptionists, etc., to look over it, and, if it might apply to them, to try answering it. Listen carefully to their feedback and comments on how it was to be a respondent. Then try it on some patients (though not those who might get it in the study proper, as this might bias the result) and get their comments. Only when all say that it is clear and easy to answer are you in a position to go onto the pilot stage of the research.

SUMMARY

This chapter has dealt principally with the process of how to devise an instrument for collecting information. The stages involved with this data-collection process are:

- consideration of qualitative as opposed to quantitative methods;
- consideration of costs and benefits between choosing a self-administered and an interview survey;
- designing a questionnaire.

SUGGESTED TASKS

1.   Design a questionnaire to measure patient satisfaction with your repeat prescription system.

2.   Design a schedule for evaluating and comparing the workload between partners.

3.   Design a questionnaire which would identify the difficulties your receptionists find with their work.

5 In the field

Previous chapters have all dealt with the theoretical principles of carrying out research. Of course in practice it is rarely as clear and logical—all sorts of things can and do go wrong. This chapter tries to give some ideas about the practical difficulties which can arise while you are 'out there' collecting data or trying to get the whole show on the road. However, the best way to learn about problems such as these is actually to meet them when doing your own research: there is no substitute for hands-on experience.

THE PILOT STUDY

A research study very rarely runs entirely smoothly, there are always unexpected problems and difficulties. The solution is to try as far as possible to anticipate, minimize, or avoid these problems, and probably the most important way of doing this is with a pilot study.

The pilot study is the dress rehearsal for the main study in which fine tuning to the practical procedures takes place. It should therefore follow as closely as possible the design of the main study, except, of course, it is carried out on a much smaller scale. The sample used should consist of people who resemble as closely as possible those who will be used in the main sample, though to prevent contamination you should not use anyone who might be included in the main study's sample. Thereafter, the data-collection procedures are run through as if this was the real research.

In an apparently straightforward study it is tempting to skimp on or ignore the pilot: don't. The best laid plans can have holes in them: you will discover that some of the questionnaire is unintelligible, the receptionists did not know that they should ask everyone a certain question, the case-numbering system did not work, your partner forgot to collect the data, you lost the random-number tables, etc. The pilot is the evidence that the practical part of the data collection will actually work; make sure that the study will work before you start the data collection proper.

The pilot study may also have an exploratory function for investigating and developing new ideas and identifying specific areas for further investigation. Sometimes this is referred to as the prepilot, it occurs prior to the pilot where the questionnaire has reached a more structured stage.

PLANNING AND PREPARATION

Preparation for the process of data collection not only involves designing an appropriate instrument for measurement but also considering and deciding upon the timetable for the data collection as well as finding and recruiting staff.

Timetabling is important in any project. Draw up a schedule at the beginning so you can keep a check on your progress. Very roughly allow about one-third of your time for planning, one-third for data collection, and one-third for analysis and writing up. For data collection you will need to timetable piloting and any printing necessary for the final questionnaire. Then you have to decide when to carry out the data collection and for how long. Occasionally these problems are inter-linked.

Question 5(1)

You want to carry out a trial of Skinnyfax with your overweight patients over four consecutive weeks. Rank the following months in terms of suitability for the project:

(a)   February;
(b)   August;
(c)   December;
(d)   October.

There is probably no ideal time. Eventually a compromise has to be reached between many factors such as:

● maximizing the likelihood of collecting the data required.
● ensuring that there is a strong likelihood of collecting a truly representative sample of the population being studied.

February tends to be a busy month in most practices and the staff would not have the time to organize and run the trial then. August would appear to be a generally quiet time—so quiet that in many practices patients and doctors go on holiday. In practices in popular holiday areas the opposite may apply—it may be the busiest time of the year with a flood of temporary residents. Either way may lead one to doubt how representative is the sample, and there may be practical difficulties associated with the collection of the data. December is a month which tends to be reasonably busy, though partners tend not to be on holiday. Unfortunately, it might not be as convenient for patients who may not have the time near Christmas to fill in a questionnaire.

It would seem that October would be a more suitable month for the project, without too many disruptions from holidays and without too much disruption to the daily functioning of the practice. However, as we have pointed out, there is no ideal time. It depends on the type of project, the type of practice, the availability of help, limitations imposed by funding bodies, etc. One can only aim for the best all-round compromise.

Similarly, when thinking about the duration of the study there are many factors to consider.

Question 5(2)

You work in a small practice and recognise that to find a sample of 300 patients (including controls) within the specified time period you will need to recruit a number of other GPs. It appears that GPs see on average one obese person every two days. How many GPs will you need to recruit to your study?

(a) 1; (b) 5; (c) 10; (d) 20; or (e) 100.

One of the major constraints on the design of any project, especially if it involves the help of other people (as it usually does), such as patients, partners, colleagues, staff, etc., will be their enthusiasm, and hence their diligence in collecting the data. On the figures you have obtained, it looks as if something like 10 overweight patients will be identified every month. Thus, in addition to yourself and your partner you would need to recruit 28 GPs to carry out the study in four weeks. Alternatively, you could extend the time period to two months and reduce the number of GPs to be recruited. Again, the compromise will be between the ability to recruit sufficient numbers of GPs who will collect the data, and the organisational problems that may be associated with collecting data from large numbers (allowing for follow-up, etc.), and recruiting a small number of GPs and expecting diligent data collection from them over what may be a long time period. You may decide that 10 GPs collecting data over a three-month period appears to be a suitable compromise. However, if you find that you cannot recruit that many GPs, you may need to rethink the design of the study, especially the sizes of the samples, rather than to extend the period of data collection from those GPs, whose enthusiasm for the project will have finite limits.

Sufficient time must also be allowed for setting up the project, last-minute administrative hitches, and for mounting the pilot study to try out your method.

Another practical problem that may occur, depending on the size of the project, is that of recruiting staff and training them. Probably for the majority of projects mounted within primary care by GPs, especially those within their own practice, this will not be a problem. The staff used in the data collection will often be the practice staff, such as receptionists, practice managers, and secretaries, adding yet another task to the many they already have. Even so, they will still need careful explanations of what is expected of them, together with the practice that the pilot study will give them.

THE PROJECT

Over coffee one day Dr Don Doolittle's attention is drawn to the fact that the female doctor in his partnership always finishes her surgery after the other partners. He therefore decides to organize and design a project to see if female GPs have longer consultations with their patients than do male GPs. He asks members of the local Young Practitioners' Group to help, but before starting he decides to run a pilot study in his own practice. He designs a form (Fig. 5.1) in which he hopes to record the length of all consultations over the course of a week.

TIME ANALYSIS FORM			
Date:		Name of GP:	
Time patient entered	Sex	Age	Time patient left

Fig. 5.1. Time analysis form.

Question 5(3)

How should he collect the information?

(a) Get his receptionist to do it.
(b) Complete it himself at the end of each consultation.
(c) Hire a clerical research helper to sit outside his room.

The preferred option is probably (b). The form is fairly simple, the information should be readily available: it just requires him to remember to do it. Hiring research staff, as in (c), to help on a fairly simple study is just not worth the time, resources, and effort, if it can be conducted by the GP in question; besides, if Dr Doolittle does it, he can keep a close eye on everything that happens.

In this instance Dr Doolittle actually decides to opt for (a), since he felt that this was a fairly simple task which the receptionist could easily fit in with her other duties. Figure 5.2 shows the completed form he received back from the receptionist. She pointed out that the start of the next consultation may not be the same as the end of the previous one, since

TIME ANALYSIS FORM			
Date:		Name of GP:	
Time patient entered	Sex	Age	Time patient left
9.03	F	30 ish	9.12
9.12	F	7	9.15
9.15	M	10	–
–	M	10	–
–	F	25	–
–	–	–	–
–	M	–	–
10.45	M	50	10.53
			Surgery ended

Fig. 5.2.   Completed time analysis form.

occasionally Dr Doolittle had odd gaps in his appointments, or makes a telephone call, and that sometimes patients can slip out without being seen. She also said that she was too busy between 9.25 and 10.20 on that Monday morning and that she had not had time to fill in the form then, but still she didn't think it would matter too much as she was sure she could remember most of the information anyway.

Question 5(4)

Should Dr Doolittle:

(a)   Decide to choose an alternative method?

(b)   Carry on regardless, since at least some of the times must be nearly right?
(c)   Sack the receptionist?

   Hopefully he should ignore options (b) and (c)! He therefore decides to fill in the form himself during surgery. He completes the first two or three satisfactorily, but then realizes half-way through the third surgery that he has not been doing it.

Question 5(5)

Should Dr Doolittle:

(a)   Try and estimate the start and finish times for the 10 patients he has seen so far?
(b)   Divide the time elapsed since surgery started by the number of patients seen to arrive during this time, and use this?
(c)   Forget about it for this surgery and hope to remember at the next?
(d)   Give himself a mental mark of 0 out of 10 for effort, and start from now?

   If he selected option (a), then probably he needs to re-read the book so far. Option (b) is probably not as daft as it sounds. The problem would be that he does not know, at this stage, what sort of analysis will be used, and whether an 'average' time is suitable—it probably is not. Also he may not allow for time not consulting, e.g. telephone calls or time spent between consultations. All in all probably best avoided.
   (c) is a perfectly safe option, but will he do any better next time? Is there not some way of ensuring that he remembers to start filling in the form at the start of the surgery—a note on his desk, a knot in his practice manager, etc.? Perhaps he can draw from this some lessons about the commitment that he is expecting from people, such as receptionists or other GPs, who have not even had the incentive of being directly involved in the planning of the project.

PROJECT NO. 2

Six months later, having completed his first project, Dr Doolittle decides to try to answer a more ambitious question: 'Would reducing the number of patients seen in surgery improve the quality of the service offered?'
   He decides to take a sample of GPs in Rawpless Health District. He sends the following letter to all 123 GPs on the medical list in that district:

                                                              Three Hats Health Centre
Dear Colleague,
   I am organizing a really interesting study into the effect of the number of patients seen in surgery on the quality of the service provided. I'm hoping to get as many

GPs as possible to take part so I hope I can count on your participation. Could you just drop me a line to let me know you are willing?

Yours sincerely,

Two weeks later he has received two replies. One is from his partner apologizing for the fact that he is on holiday in the near future and so will not be able to take part. The other is from a 60-year-old, single-handed, ex-member of the GMSC who demands to know whether he is in the pay of the 'CHC or some other leftie group'.

Question 5(6)

Should Dr Doolittle now:

(a) Carry on with himself as his sample?
(b) Decide to ask the trainers at the next trainers' workshop to take part?
(c) Approach the local GP-subcommittee or LMC for their support?

Option (b) is a commonly practised ploy for those hoping to attract GPs who are in some way more committed, or likely to be keener about being involved in research projects. Similarly, Dr Doolittle might consider approaching college members or young practitioner groups. The two main problems are:

1. There is no guarantee that these groups will be any more amenable to persuasion than the larger groups, especially if the method of persuasion is as impersonal as before.
2. The more highly selected the subgroup, the less Dr Doolittle would be able to generalize from his findings to the larger group. His population becomes 'GPs who are trainers in Rawpless' and not 'all GPs in Rawpless'.

The best option is probably (c). However, Dr Doolittle might have to rethink his approach. Rather than an impersonal letter, it may be more politic to go and see the clerk of the LMC, or the Chairman of the GP subcommittee and suggest that the project may help to show indirectly that if list sizes were reduced so as to make surgeries smaller then services to patients might be improved, etc.

Question 5(7)

Which of the following bodies might it be appropriate to approach for their views and co-operation?

(a) Family Practitioner Committee;
(b) District Health Authority;
(c) District Ethical Committee;
(d) Local Medical Committee;

(e)   Consultant Medical Advisory Committee;
(f)   Community Health Council;
(g)   Medical Defence Union.

As with so many of the practical aspects of planning a project, one is faced with problems, the solutions to which may interfere with each other. In this case, one wants to gain the confidence and co-operation of parties representing those likely to be affected by the project in order to increase the response rate, yet one does not want this stage of the planning to drag on interminably while the views of committee after committee are sought.

If Dr Doolittle was surveying a large group of GPs in a district, it would make sense to take his plans to any representative body that might exist, such as an LMC or GP subcommittee. Similarly with the consultants. If the number to be solicited is small, then personal discussion is the best method of achieving co-operation. If the number is larger, he should seek out a representative body for their views, such as the relevant Medical Advisory Committee. The Community Health Council might be thought to be at least one body which represents the patients at a group. It is doubtful whether any project needs to be referred to bodies such as DHAs, FPCs, or MDUs. (Though he might want the advice or co-operation of individuals, such as the District Medical Officer or FPC Administrator, within such organizations.)

Within the practice setting, as we have mentioned above, it is just as important to spend time and effort getting peoples' co-operation. If there is a Patient Participation Group in the practice, perhaps they could be used as a source of opinion about the methodology chosen. Time spent in ensuring the co-operation of those helping with the data collection, both collectors and respondents, will be amply rewarded in increasing the response rate from the project and so helping to ensure the adequacy of the sample taken.

Dr Doolittle therefore sees the chairman of the local LMC to elicit his support. Dr Doolittle explains to him that he would like to choose 20 GPs from Rawpless Health District randomly, contact them, and persuade them to take part in his study. He points out the earlier published work suggesting that a longer time spent with a patient improves patient care, and suggests that if he could show that reducing the number of patients seen per surgery session, irrespective of the time spent with each patient, would improve the service provided, then that would be a strong argument for a reduction in individual list size. The chairman seems very interested but before agreeing to take the matter further asks whether Dr Doolittle has been through the ethical committee.

Question 5(8)

Should Dr Doolittle:

(a)   Disagree that it needs to be referred to them?
(b)   Agree to immediately refer the project to his local ethical committee?

Option (a) is not likely to please the chairman, and therefore Dr Doolittle might put his co-operation at risk. However, it does have the advantage of reducing the time-scale. There could be a compromise. Option (b) is the correct course, but could be very time-consuming. The design does not directly affect patient care, so it may be sufficient to discuss the project with the chairman of the local ethical committee.

The chairman of the ethical committee agrees that there are no serious ethical considerations, and that Dr Doolittle can proceed, but he requests a protocol which he will put before the committee when it next meets. (And since Dr Doolittle is obviously so keen on research, and as there is a vacancy on the ethical committee for the token GP, he invites him to be a member of that committee.)

ETHICAL CONSIDERATIONS

On the basis that any interaction with patients has the potential for harm, probably all projects involving patient opinions or details should be referred automatically to the local ethical committee. However, it is a matter for judgement, and in the not-too-distant past (and possibly the present in some areas) the make-up of these committees had little to do with the type of research commonly carried out in general practice. The 'District Ethical Committee' was often a subcommittee of the hospital consultants' committee structure, and almost entirely composed of this species of animal, who, if certain stories are to be believed, seemed more content to allow a double-blind trial than a question to patients about what their doctors told them. However, times are changing, and these committees are becoming far more broadly based in their composition, with representation from many groups, including hospital consultants, GPs, and Community Health Councils. As well as being an important step in its own right, in that it may draw attention to aspects of planning that may have slipped 'unnoticed' into the design of a project, it is often necessary to obtain such approval in any projects for which outside funding is being sought, especially when patients are involved.

It should be possible to trace the whereabouts of your local ethical committee either through your postgraduate centre or library, or through the District Health Authority.

Question 5(9)

As a member of the local medical ethical committee, Dr Doolittle has received the following protocol for a research project. What comments should he make on it, and how might it be changed to improve its chances of ethical committee approval?

Research protocol

Title: Assessing the effect of vitamin B on the hypersensitivity of bronchial smooth muscle in primates.

It is hypothesized that hypovitaminosis may lead to a potentiation of the bronchial smooth muscles, and that eliminating such deficiencies will lessen the sensitivity of the musculature to external stimuli.

Aim: It is the aim of the project to assess the effect of regular vitamin B supplements on the peak-flow readings of people known to have bronchial hypersensitivity.

Problem: The null hypothesis can be stated as: Daily supplements of vitamin B will not cause a significant increase in the early morning peak-flow readings.

Details of method: Since asthma is common in young people it is proposed to look at people aged 1–10 years, known to have bronchial hypersensitivity. A sample of these patients will be identified from the discharge summaries of a district general hospital. No further prescriptions for anti-asthmatic treatment will be issued for a period of two weeks leading to the start of the trial, to allow base-line values of peak flow to be established. Families and GPs of the patients will be sent an explanatory letter. The sample will be divided into an intervention and a control group, matched for age and sex. The intervention group will be given vitamin B tablets, two daily, for two weeks, and the control group a placebo. Early morning peak flows will be measured in both groups. Withdrawal from the trial will be solely at the discretion of the project director, to whom application should be made.

Application: It is expected that the results will provide interesting and valuable information on the role of vitamin B on the Zartolf–Baronsky receptors in the bronchial musculature of primates.

When choosing groups to study, special care should be taken with:

(1)   children;
(2)   unemployed;
(3)   prisoners;
(4)   pregnant women;
[(5)   solicitors.]

Some groups are easier to identify, e.g. pregnant women, or to study, e.g. prisoners. However, it is important that the vulnerability of the group be considered. Most patients trust their doctors, and may well consent to almost any proposal. It goes without saying that the doctor carries a moral responsibility for actions that are, or are not, proposed. This is more obvious in a clinical trial type of project, but may be equally important in attitudinal surveys. For pregnant women, infants, and children under 10, the requirements for informed consent should be particularly stringent, and the method to be used for obtaining consent should be clearly indicated. Similarly, the benefits that are likely to accrue from their involvement in research projects should be made clear to groups such as prisoners, and their informed consent obtained. In the protocol above, one needs to ask 'Why children?' In any research using children as the study population, one should ask, 'Can this study be carried out only on children?'

Question 5(10)

Involvement in a research project should, where possible, be preceded by:

(a) nothing;
(b) verbal explanation;
(c) written explanation;
(d) verbal consent;
(e) written consent.

As we have said, patients, for some reason, tend to trust their doctor. It therefore means that the doctor should do everything to ensure that this trust is neither damaged nor misplaced. The words 'informed consent' implies a range of meaning, and probably hides a multitude of sins. The method of informing the patient about the project and their involvement in it, and then seeking their consent, will obviously vary with the type, complexity, and implied risk of the project. The important point is that the problem must be considered properly and carefully, and an ethical committee will be looking very carefully at this part of a protocol. In the example above, there was no attempt to seek consent at any level from the parents. 'A letter of explanation' was to be sent. Yet the design of the trial was such as to put a vulnerable group, children and especially asthmatic children, at considerable risk.

Question 5(11)

Withdrawal from a project should be at the discretion of:

(a) the patient;
(b) the project director;
(c) the patient's doctor;
(d) the ethical committee.

The withdrawal from a project of any type, at any stage, must remain the right of the patient. Similarly, any doctor must remain free to remove a patient under his or her care from a project, especially a trial, or to give additional treatment at any time, if it seems to be in the patient's best interests. In the example, withdrawal from a dangerous trial was to be at the discretion of the project director—an obviously unrealistic and unethical approach.

In summary, it is important to consider the ethical issues implicit on the design of any project. One needs to ask:

1.   Is the research necessary? Will it have positive applications for future health care?

2.   Will the research project be well planned and executed? It is unethical to carry out any project that is not.

There were considerable misgivings a few years ago about a number of so-called 'drug trials' whereby GPs were paid on a per capita basis to start patients on various treatments, e.g. a course of an antihypertensive agent. The patient was then to be followed up over a number of months and an assessment made of efficacy, side-effects, etc. Many thought that these trials were unethical in that they were unnecessary, the efficacy of the drug was already known from earlier studies, and the studies themselves were poorly designed in that they were neither 'blind' nor 'controlled'. Several opinions were voiced that the whole event was a method of soft-selling, and that at the end of the 'trial' the only outcome was that the company had achieved a market share for their product and that many GPs had been misled into believing that they had been involved in 'research'.

3.   If the trial or product involves children, is it of such a nature that it can only be carried out on children?

4.   Has the informed consent of the patient, or the parent, been obtained, before their participation and before randomization?

5.   Is it clear that patients are free to withdraw from the trial at any time if they so wish?

6.   Is it clear that any doctor responsible for the care of the patient is free to remove that patient from the trial, or to give additional treatment at any time, if he or she feels it to be in the patient's best interest?

7.   Is the project to be controlled and supervised by a properly constituted ethical committee?

Hopefully this has given you some idea of the areas covered by ethical considerations of projects and trials. The WHO has produced the *Helsinki Declaration* on the subject, the main points of which can be found in a medical library.

Dr Doolittle returns to the problem of finding 20 doctors to take part in his plan. The chairman of the LMC is also now satisfied and so he selects a random sample of 20 GPs from the medical list for Rawpless.

Question 5(12)

The chairman of the LMC suggests to Dr Doolittle that he should send a joint letter to these doctors asking them to participate.
  Should Dr Doolittle agree?

  Yes? Despite the extra weight of the LMC sanction, a written request is likely to have little more success than the initial letter.
  No? Dr Doolittle tactfully suggests that the LMC chairman writes a letter which he can then show the GPs when he visits them to explain the project, and to try and persuade them to participate.
  Using a table of random numbers and the local medical list, Dr Doolittle identifies his sample of 20 doctors. He makes appointments to see them all, and explains the outline of the project, why they have been chosen, the backing of the local LMC, and the likely consequences from the results.

Question 5(13)

Despite this, eight of the 20 decide not to take part. Should Dr Doolittle:

(a) Accuse them of anti-social behaviour and report them to the GMC?
(b) Make up the number from among his own partners, trainees, and colleagues?
(c) Take another eight names from the list using the list of random numbers, and contact these as before?

  Option (a) has its appeal, but probably sticking pins into effigies is just as effective. Option (b) would mean that the sample was no longer random. However, with eight out of 20 refusing to take part, for whatever reason, there are going to be doubts about the randomness of the sample whichever method is chosen. This is probably not the best alternative, though it may be the most practical.
  Option (c) is probably the best thing to do. However, based on the previous drop-out rate, only four of these may be willing to take part, and it may be that by the time 20 places have been filled Dr Doolittle will have approached almost half his possible population, with all the appointments and visiting that this approach will entail.

Question 5(14)

What should Dr Doolittle do about the drop-outs?

(a) Ignore them as unscientific doctors.
(b) Record information about them for future use!

  Much as Dr Doolittle would like to, he cannot ignore them as there may be something different about this sizeable subgroup, besides their non-compliance to research invitations. Option (b) may appear to contain a touch of 'big brother', but in fact Dr Doolittle will need to know whether this group of non-responders differed in any way from his responding GPs. That is, was there anything different about them which may affect the extent to which the final sample will reflect the characteristics of all the doctors in Rawpless. To that end he will need to record the characteristics of his non-responders to compare them with his responders in the analysis.

INTERVIEWING

Dr Sophie Middleyear decides to look at the connection between symptoms associated with the so-called 'male' as well as female menopause, and life events. She designs a questionnaire to be put to a sample of her patients aged between 40 and 55. She feels that an interview will be a more effective way of eliciting information than a postal questionnaire, but because of resource limitations she has to carry out some of the interviewing herself. Although she has never done any interviewing before, she does not envisage any problems. After all, she spends most of her day talking to patients and interviewing is only a matter of establishing and recording the information she needs. So off she goes to find some patients, with a bunch of questionnaires in her hand, and a pencil behind her ear.

But hold on. How does she find a sample of respondents? In Chapter 2 we saw that random sampling should enable her to limit the size of her project without necessarily affecting the meaningfulness of her results. Therefore she identifies the 50 names and addresses of a sample of 40–55-year-old patients from the practice age–sex register. She has a young trainee who is keen to help her. How does she decide which patients should be interviewed by which interviewer?

Question 5(15)

Should Dr Middleyear pick out:

(a) Patients whom she knows will be friendly?
(b) Patients who live in certain affluent areas because she finds poorer people a bit stroppy?
(c) Male patients as she finds female patients a bit difficult?
(d) All patients in a certain area?

All interviewers should try to interview a cross-section of the sample, so options (a) and (b) should not be used. However, there are limitations on time and resources, and it would seem wise to allocate addresses in the same locality to each interviewer.

The first name on Dr Middleyear's list is:

> Mrs Olive Wintergreen,
> 83 The Walk,
> Little Puddle-on-Sea.

Her knock is answered by a Mr Biggs who tells her that Mrs Wintergreen no longer lives there.

Question 5(16)

Should Dr Middleyear:

(a) Finish the interview there and then?
(b) Interview Mr Biggs?
(c) Ask for Mrs Wintergreen's new address?

Option (c) is the usual course of action, and a decision has to be made about how far movers should be followed up. However, some studies use a substituting procedure where a substitute is picked. This is acceptable so long as the randomness of the sample is not compromised.

The next name and address on her list is:

> Mr A. Daly,
> Warrick Mansion,
> The Hill,
> Little Puddle-on-Sea.

When Dr Middleyear gets there she gets no reply and the house looks suspiciously vacant and derelict.

Question 5(17)

Should she:

(a) Ask the neighbours where Mr Daly has moved to?
(b) Call back later, just in case he is out?
(c) Give up and send a postal questionnaire?

Occasionally the house will be derelict or vacant. Interviewers can then make enquiries with neighbours, to find out where the occupants have moved to. On other occasions the respondents will just be out at the time the interviewer calls. In such cases the interviewer will usually make up to three visits before a decision is made to give up the attempt at gaining an interview.

Obtaining an interview

Disheartened, Dr Middleyear wonders if she should have done a project on housing. Where is everyone? She moves onto the third name and address on her list hoping for more luck.

> Mrs Pamela Croucher,
> 2, Battle Drive,
> Greater Puddle-on-Sea.

Eureka! The lady in question is at home. So Dr Middleyear gives her the basic information about the survey, its relevance and why she has been selected. Despite this she seems very reluctant to take part.

Question 5(18)

Should Dr Middleyear:

(a)   Give up and accept the refusal?
(b)   Tell her that she is being uncooperative and threaten to strike her off her list?
(c)   Gently persuade her to take part?

One of the most difficult but crucial steps is to get the respondent to agree to be interviewed. Increasingly people are wary of strangers appearing at their homes and asking them to divulge information about their private lives. Obviously option (b) should never be used because every respondent has the right to refuse, and it is up to the interviewer to put a reasonable case rather than to tell the respondent that he or she is in some way morally wrong not to take part in this vitally important research. Obviously much will depend on the strength of the respondent's feelings about being interviewed, and it may be that giving up and accepting the refusal is the right course. However, in some cases gentle persuasion is possible.

Question 5(19)

Spend a few minutes thinking of the points that could be made in an attempt to gently persuade Mrs Croucher to take part.

It may purely be a question of convenience—offering to return at a more convenient time may be all that is needed. It could be that she does not fully understand why she has been picked out (Is there something wrong with her?), and so emphasizing the random structure of the sampling and her selection, and fully and clearly explaining the importance of gaining an interview with her, may help her to change her mind. It may be that she doesn't know who the interviewer is, and this may be the case especially if other helpers are used—some form of identification might help. Some of this uncertainty can be overcome by sending a letter to the sample prior to commencing the study, telling them about the study and asking for their co-operation. The respondent then has the option of contacting the researcher directly to find out more about the study or to refuse to take part, thereby not wasting travelling time. However, sending a letter has the danger of encouraging refusals and, in general, face-to-face contact between interviewer and respondent is a better way of gaining co-operation than by more formal means such as a letter.

Asking the questions

Pamela eventually lets Dr Middleyear in. She settles down with a cup of tea to ask the questions. After the first few questions it becomes clear that Mrs Croucher's responses, particularly with the open-ended questions, are unclear, incomplete, and irrelevant.

Question 5(20)

Should Dr Middleyear:

(a)   Accept what is said and write it down verbatim?
(b)   Ignore the unclear replies and move onto the next question?
(c)   Avoid and omit open-ended questions?
(d)   Clarify the answer for the respondent?
(e)   Allow for an expectant pause?
(f)   Encourage a response, e.g. 'that's interesting?'
(g)   Repeat the question?
(h)   Use a supplementary question or probe for clarification: 'I'm not quite sure what you mean?'
(i)   Add neutral comments such as 'anything else?'

Options (d) to (i) are accepted procedures used by trained interviewers to elicit full responses to questions. Thus it may be helpful to sit down with any helpers, before starting, to go over the questions and their meanings. This may also be the time to point out that the success from such interviews can also depend on the tone of voice, manner, gesture, and personal characteristics of the interviewer, as well as the circumstances under which the interview is carried out. Depending on the type and subject matter of the questions, it might be possible to maximize the success of the survey by recruiting helpers to interview according to age, social class, gender, etc.

After three hours with Mrs Croucher and with only three of the 46 questions answered—and for two of those the still confused replies were only extracted after the shedding of much blood, sweat, and tears—Dr Middleyear decides to pass over this part of the project totally to her trainee.

CONFIDENTIALITY AND DATA PROTECTION

Research projects involve the collection and analysis of some form of data. Research of health-care issues invariably involves information about individuals, whether they be patients, doctors, or other health-care workers. This information may be about the individuals or may consist of their opinions about various issues. Much of it will only be given freely by that individual if they are convinced about the confidentiality of their contributions. Confidentiality can be threatened both in the collection and in the analysis of the research data. Often confidentiality can be put at risk, unbeknown to the patients concerned, through the research method chosen.

Dr John Batter has decided to analyse the effect of intervention by the health visitor in families in which it is suspected a non-accidental injury has occurred to a child. A review of the families' medical records is undertaken to assess subsequent health problems in members of these families.

Question 5(21)

Who should Dr Batter ask to search the records to record the information?

(a)   The practice secretary;
(b)   The temporarily attached research worker;
(c)   The practice-attached health visitor;
(d)   The GP.

It is common knowledge, and indeed common practice in these days of primary health-care teams, to find that access to patients' records is not totally and absolutely restricted to the patient's doctor. In the daily running of a practice the notes are handled by an assortment of clerks, receptionists, secretaries, nurses, health visitors, etc. Running a research project that involves the perusal of patient records lays open these records to more people, with resultant loss of confidentiality. Even if the subject matter is not as sensitive as in the example here, a search through records for any reason may reveal information that was only given initially on the assumption that doctor–patient confidentiality was assured. Such searches should, in an ideal world, only be undertaken by the doctor. However, once again economy of time and effort may demand less than the ideal, and any resulting compromise should be arrived at only after the most careful consideration of aspects of confidentiality. Similar problems in the data-collection part of the research may follow from the use of non-medical assistants to conduct face-to-face interviews, especially with clinicians. Many clinicians, and indeed ethical committees, are extremely wary about the use of such helpers in the collection of what may be sensitive opinions or facts.

Having collected the data there are still problems of confidentiality in the method chosen to store the data. This method will obviously depend in part on what resources are available. However, the ultimate object of the exercise is to analyse the data so as to answer the question that was originally proposed. This will be discussed in greater depth in Chapter 6, but here it is necessary to point out that thought needs to be given to the relative confidentiality of the methods available.

A great pile of scraps of paper will obviously not be easy to analyse, and the degree of confidentiality this affords will be dependent on the ability to keep the scraps together, and to prevent unauthorized access to them.

Computerized data-bases are nowadays extremely common and available. They are relatively easy to use, both to store the data in whatever way is required, and to allow it to be presented in a form suitable for analysis. However, they are perceived by both public and now government as being considerably less than perfect in protecting the confidentiality of data about individuals. It is too easy to ask a computer, if it in fact stores such details, to produce a list of one-legged, homosexuals working as security officers in the north-west of Scotland. Newspaper stories of computer enthusiasts 'hacking' their way into Prince Philip's private computer mailbox, or into the Pentagon's main computer have somewhat dented faith in the various 'password' methods that are meant to protect computer-held information from unauthorized, prying eyes.

The Data Protection Act requires anyone who is storing patient details electronically to register their use of a computer for this purpose. Universities and research institutes will be able to advise you on this but as they will probably already have a 'blanket' registration under the Act you may be able to carry out your research under the aegis of such arrangements. Besides, you may well be using university/medical school computing for your analysis (as described in a later chapter).

Probably the practical compromise most commonly used in data storage is to keep the 'raw' but sensitive data in some manual but systematic paper file. A card-index file or a loose-leaf folder, with one card or page for each 'subject', usually allows the data to be easily transcribed onto a coding frame for computer analysis, yet by being a relatively compact method of storage does permit measures to be taken to maximize confidentiality.

SUMMARY

This chapter has attempted to look at various practical considerations concerned in the carrying out of any project. Although we have tried to stress that doing research, of whatever complexity, can be extremely rewarding and enjoyable, it does require the use of resources. It is therefore extremely important that these resources are used efficiently and effectively. The major resource will be your energy.

There will be times in most projects when you wonder if the problems which have cropped up are not insuperable: that is the point when you will have to show patience and perseverance. And of course by careful planning, in the form of a clearly presented research design and a rigorous pilot study, you should minimize these difficulties.

Remember that probably the most precious resources, which need to be nurtured and treated with great consideration, are the patients, colleagues, partners, and staff whose co-operation you will be seeking, not just for the present project, but possibly again in the not-too-distant future.

SUGGESTED TASK

Find out the composition and procedures of your Local Ethical Committee. How often does it meet? What percentage of applications are turned down, or are requested to be changed?

6 Data into numbers

Chapter 4 described how data could be collected and Chapter 5 dealt with some of the practical difficulties of actually doing that collecting. It is now time to retire to your inner sanctum excitedly clutching your data. Analysis! Results! Publications! An OBE?

But look at your data: a pile of questionnaires? A collection of tape cassettes? A jumble of field notes? How are these to be analysed to produce those heady 'results'? This chapter examines the first stage in that process for quantitative studies, namely the process by which newly collected data is transformed into numbers.

A NOTE ON QUALITATIVE METHODS

Chapter 4 outlined the overall process of collecting specific data from the mass of data 'out there'. These data could be collected by unstructured, semi-structured, and structured means, and each of these forms of data require different treatments to enable analysable results to emerge.

Some unstructured data can be analysed without recourse to numbers. Interviews with patients on the meanings they ascribe to their illnesses, for example, might be analysed in terms of the variety and types of meaning system used. Certainly this form of data could be converted into numbers—as we shall see—but almost inevitably with some loss of quality. Although analysing numbers is the traditional way of doing research, it is increasingly recognized that if we are aiming to reach a deeper understanding of things, qualitative studies have an important role to play. A structured questionnaire of receptionists' views of patients might give some numbers to play with, but a few in-depth interviews may reveal far more of interest than would 1000 fixed-format questionnaires.

This chapter concentrates on quantitative research but this is not to imply that it is necessarily superior. It all depends on what you are trying to do. If your research question is about whether winter-born children are more likely to develop URTIs during the rest of their childhoods, you must have a quantitative study. But if you want to know how the children's parents cope with these infections, you might find a qualitative study of greater value. We understand very little about general practice and so different approaches all have an important part to play.

QUANTITATIVE STUDIES

Let us first take an overview of the rest of the research process after data collection.

- data are converted into numbers;
- numbers will need to be analysed by manipulation (Chapter 7) or by statistical tests (Chapter 8);
- results will be written up (Chapter 9).

The analysis will probably be carried out using a computer, either a large computer (or 'mainframe' as it is called) as is found in universities— gaining access by a 'terminal'—or by a stand-alone personal computer (as might be found in a general practice) using a statistical software package. Details of these come later. Whichever method of data analysis is available, we shall need to present our data in a form that makes it easy to analyse.

THE DATA-FILE

Computers need to 'read' numbers in an assimilable form: this form is the 'data-file' (a 'file' being a discrete collection of information stored in a computer, analogous to a file in a filing cabinet).

Dr Verity Tally is interested in exploring the patterns of work in her consultations. She collects data on all the patients she sees during a week, together with information on whether she wrote a prescription or referred for investigation or an out-patient appointment. She sees 130 patients in the week and collects the relevant data on a schedule, in the form of an audit sheet, which she designed specially for the purpose. She then processes her data into a data-file, the first five lines of which look like this:

$$0016922111$$
$$0025411112$$
$$0034322111$$
$$0042321111$$
$$0053212211$$

What does it all mean? Fortunately Dr Tally knows, and she will let the computer into the secret so that it too can 'read' the data-file.

The data-file is a series of columns running downwards, and rows running across. Looking down the left hand three columns you should be able to see a pattern. Each set of three digits is a number, ascending from one line to the next. This is because each line or row represents one 'case'—in this instance one patient who was seen by Dr Tally in her survey week. In this example each case is 10 digits long but in other studies it might be longer or shorter, depending on how much data on each has been collected (statistical packages tend to cope with a maximum line length of 80 digits, but each case can, if needed, take up several lines).

Let us explore what each line means. Take the first one:

0016922111

Although it might look like either ten separate numbers or as one large one, it is in fact several groups of numbers. In this example Dr Tally knows that the digits break up into the following groups:

001 69 2 2 1 1 1

The first three columns contain the case number. In this instance it is 001. The case number requires three digits because, as you will recall, Dr Tally collected 130 patients in her audit. Had she collected a sample of 9 or less, then one column would have sufficed; on the other hand, if her sample had been over 999, then she would have required four columns/digits, the first case becoming 0001.

The next two columns contain the patient's age. This is very straightforward. It is clear that the first patient was 69; equally, going back to the data-file we can see the second patient was aged 54, and so on.

Dr Tally reserved the sixth column for the patient's sex. A '2'? Dr Tally started off with two possibilities, male or female. But the computer does not read words as part of the English language so Dr Tally has to devise a *code* to represent the two sexes to the computer. The code could be groups of letters such as 'MALE' or 'FEMALE' but this is rather cumbersome as well as wasteful. The more usual way of coding is to assign one number to each category. In this case Dr Tally chose: male = 1; female = 2. Thus, knowing the code, we can see that the first patient she recorded was a 69-year-old female.

In similar fashion the next four columns are reserved for codes of practice activity. The coding system which Dr Tally chose was as under:

Column 7	Prescription	no = 1
		yes = 2
Column 8	X-ray?	no = 1
		yes = 2
Column 9	Pathology?	no = 1
		yes = 2
Column 10	OP referral?	no = 1
		yes = 2

Now, reading along the data line we can see that the first patient in the audit was a 69-year-old woman who received a prescription but was not referred for an X-ray, pathology investigation, or to out-patients.

It all begins to make sense. Which patient was referred to out-patients?

The second, because there is a figure '2' in the tenth column. Which was the youngest patient to receive a prescription? The fifth, who was aged 32. (The fourth was the youngest at 23 but the figure '1' in the sixth column, indicates that no prescription was issued.)

For a small number of cases (or small 'data-set', as the technical term has it) the data-file can be read 'manually'. However, with the full data-file of 130 cases, reading this sort of data off visually becomes a chore, even more so with hundreds of cases and perhaps 80 columns of data for each. But this sort of task is precisely what computers are good at. So long as the computer knows the code it can read off whatever information we require. Moreover, the computer can manipulate the data. It can be asked, for example, to add all the ages and divide by the number of cases to produce an average (mean) age. It can calculate the percentage of patients receiving prescriptions by adding the 2s in column seven and expressing the result as a percentage of all the cases. And, more interestingly, it can compare some cases with others: are women, for instance, more likely to receive prescriptions than men? (Which are the women? Read column six. Which of those received prescriptions? Read column seven. Compare this result with the figures for men, etc.)

This manipulation of numbers in the data-file will be more fully explored in the next two chapters. Suffice it to say that computers can, at our command, carry out elaborate analyses with data-files. Our task for the moment, however, is to translate our collected data in such a format. How is this done? Basically it depends on how categorized our collected data are already. The simplest type of data to transform into a data-file is 'structured' data, while the most complicated is 'unstructured'. (The broad outlines of why this is so were given in Chapter 4.) Let us start with the easier task: structured data.

STRUCTURED SCHEDULES

Chapter 4 described three types of structured schedule, namely a clinical schedule, an extraction schedule, and a traditional questionnaire. There was a similar format in all of these:

$$\text{closed question} \rightarrow \boxed{\text{answer}}$$

A series of closed questions were answered by the respondent or researcher in fixed format. We know the answer format is relatively fixed because the closed question ensured this was so. We can reasonably assume that a question about height in metres will not be answered in terms of weight, or, hopefully, in units other than metres.

The task of transforming responses into numbers is therefore a relatively straightfoward one. The pile of questionnaires/schedules has to be *coded*, that is the set responses have to be transcribed into numbers and entered into a data-file as described above.

Let us look at some general points about coding. The process goes like this:

$$\text{Responses on schedule} \rightarrow \text{Numbers on data sheet} \rightarrow \text{Data file in computer}$$

The traditional way of transforming numbers into the computer was by first 'punching' holes at appropriate places on a special data-card using a special sort of typewriter. Each case had a separate card. These cards were then 'read' by a machine and the data automatically entered into the computer. With the advent of the personal computer this process has been shortened by typing the numbers not onto a card but directly into the computer using the number key-pad usually found on standard computer keyboards. Even so, although numbers are now entered directly, the old expression of 'punching' data is still used to describe this process.

Punching large quantities of data into a computer can be a chore and, if your data is extensive, you might find it worthwhile to pay to have it done by technicians who are as fast at typing numbers as secretaries are at typing letters. (Ask about this facility at your local University Department of General Practice.) If you do want to do it yourself, you will need to use the 'editor' which comes with your personal computer (EDLIN is the MSDOS standard one). Possibly easier, if you have wordprocessor software, is either to type the numbers in as an 'unformatted' document or get the programme to create an ASCII file. This can be read as a data-file by either statistical software you might use yourself or by the software used by more complex mainframe computers.

Coding formats

How do we code Dr Tally's audit? In part it depends on how she recorded her data. Let us look at two formats she might have used.

Number	Age	Sex	Prescription	X-ray	Path.	OP·
001	69	F				
002	54	M				
003	43	F				

This format, which records all the data onto one sheet, might need some intermediate steps before it is punched. This might be a 'data-sheet' which involves writing down on a separate sheet of paper the appropriate numbers based on the coding frame described earlier. The endpoint would be a handwritten data-file, which would then be punched onto the computer.

The alternative—as the data is relatively straightforward—is to punch it in directly, doing the coding as you read the original data. Thus you might run your finger along one line of data, code it in your head, and punch it out on the keyboard with your other hand. This technique cuts out the separate data-sheet step and would therefore seem more efficient. However, you are likely to have to do the punching yourself as the trained 'punchers' tend to work only from data-sheets. (Quite reasonably they cannot be expected to memorize the proper codings for every piece of research they punch in.)

The other common format in which to collect data is to have a separate sheet for every case. In Dr Tally's project it might look like this:

Audit sheet

Number	☐ ☐ ☐
Age	☐ ☐
Sex (M/F)	☐
Prescription	☐
X-ray	☐
Pathology	☐
OP referral	☐

Here again, as with the earlier example, data can be directly punched or first transcribed onto a data-sheet. There is, however, a short-cut to the latter procedure because the space on the schedule allows us to place the 'data-sheet' on the same piece of paper. Thus:

Audit sheet

		For office use only
Number	☐ ☐ ☐	
Age	☐ ☐	
Sex (M/F)	☐	
Prescription	☐	
X-ray	☐	
Pathology	☐	
OP referral	☐	

A margin is poached down the right-hand side of the paper and bears a threatening title such as 'Office use only' or 'Please do not write in this margin'. The reason for keeping it clear is to allow the actual numbers for the data-file to be written in. Moreover, the boxes for the data-file numbers can be annotated with the numbers of the column in which the data is to be entered. (Though notice that boxes/columns 1–5 do not require transcribing as the researcher/respondent enters the actual number directly onto the schedule.) This way, especially when there are lots of data per case, the puncher can keep an accurate check on which column each digit goes into.

The final piece of the jigsaw is for the 'coder' to have a 'coding sheet' describing the numbers which will represent whatever answers are on the sheet. In Dr Tally's project it might looking something like this:

Coding sheet for audit

Columns

1–3	Number
4–5	Age
6	Sex: male = 1; female = 2
7	Prescription ⎱
8	X-ray ⎰ no = 1
9	Pathology ⎰ yes = 2
10	OP referral ⎰

If each member of her family has a pen and a coding sheet, Dr Tally would be able to pile her schedules on the kitchen table and quickly 'code' her 130 cases.

Coding rules

There are several conventions in coding, none of which are vital to follow, but which show good sense and order; you may like to copy them.

Make the actual number the code

In Dr Tally's coding sheet she did not give a separate code for the case number. She could have, of course. It would have been possible to multiply the patient's number by three and use that number: possible but silly. Clearly the sensible thing with many numbers is to code them directly: height, weight, diastolic pressure, etc. can all be punched intact.

Categorize clumsy numbers or ones in which precision is doubtful

Patient's height (metres) | 1.4847 |

Sometimes the researcher or the respondent gives too much detail. A height given to a fraction of a millimetre is not worth coding complete unless the research was particularly concerned with very fine variations in height. The customary technique in science is to 'round up or down'. This, in fact, is a sort of categorization because if we decide we only want height to the nearest centimetre then the coding rule is:

$$1.4650–1.4749 = 1.47$$
$$1.4750–1.4849 = 1.48$$
$$1.4850–1.4949 = 1.49$$

In this case our example would be coded as 1.48 as it falls into this category.

This principle can be extended to group any kind of data we get. For example, Dr Tally coded age as the actual age in years. She might, however, have decided that she was only interested in ten-year age bands and thus her coding rule might have looked like this:

under 20 = 1
20–29 = 2
30–39 = 3
40–49 = 4
50–59 = 5
60–69 = 6
over 69 = 7

Using this schema her first patient, the 69-year-old woman would have scored '7' for her age (and Dr Tally would have needed one column fewer in her data-file).

Alternatively, Dr Tally might only have been interested in her elderly population. She could thus have devised a dichotomous scale:

under 65 = 1
65 and over = 2

Her first patient would then have scored '2'. Clearly, the categories employed will depend on the precise research question, and the coding scheme for age in one study might be completely inappropriate for another. A word of caution though. Dr Tally might have started out being interested in her prescribing rate amongst her elderly compared with that amongst her younger patients, and therefore coded either 1 or 2 for age. However, if she finds higher prescribing amongst her elderly and wonders whether perhaps there is a linear relationship between age and prescribing, such that the older you are the more prescriptions you get, she cannot test this on her data: remember, she 'lost' her precise age data by only coding it '1' or '2'. A wiser course of action—if resources and space permit—is to code numbers as completely as possible. Dr Tally could then ask the computer to split her sample into 'young' and 'elderly' and, if she wants to go back to the original ages, she can ask the computer to unsplit them again into their original ages as given in the data-file.

Coding non-integer data

Much of the collected data are likely to be in a dichotomous scale, e.g. drug/not drug, consulted/not consulted, and here a simple 1/2 will suffice as the code. Other data will be in the form of a number which can be transcribed as outlined above. Yet other data will have no clear mathematical transformation and in these cases codes can be assigned arbitrarily.

Protestant = 1
Catholic   = 2
Jew   = 3
Other   = 4

Thus religious affiliation might be coded as above; or it might be coded 4, 3, 2, 1 or 3, 1, 2, 4. It really doesn't matter. So long as particular religious groups are coded consistently with the same code number and the computer is told what that code is then it can all be sorted out later.

Missing answers, don't knows, spoiled replies

Not infrequently, especially in self-administered questionnaires, data are incomplete. Respondents might simply omit to answer a question; or they might answer it 'inappropriately'. Sometimes whole questionnaires have to be rejected because of this and the respondent placed in the non-response category, as if they had declined to take part in the study. Often, however, some questions are answered appropriately but others need to be coded after a little thought.

Question 6(1)

How would you code the following responses?

(a) Are you male or female?   male ☐ *cheeky!*
     (Please tick)   female ☐
(b) Are you male or female?   male ☐
     (Please tick)   female ☐
(c) Are you male or female?   male ☐
     (Please tick)   female ☐ *woman*
(d) Are you male or female?   male ☒
     (Please tick)   female ☐

(a) Not the most helpful of respondents. In a survey of transsexuals we might take this response seriously and give it its own code, say 3, but in this instance it would count as a spoiled answer and, following a common convention which reserves '9' for missing answers, we code it '9'.

(b) The question was simply not answered. It cannot therefore be coded either 1 or 2 and must be scored as missing, with a 9.

(c) Not answered precisely as we requested but it would seem reasonable to code this respondent as female, 2.

(d) We asked for a tick in the appropriate box but here 'male' was marked with a cross. Was the cross a substitute for a tick? Or does it signify 'not' male? We cannot know. But perhaps if we look at the other responses in the questionnaire we can decide whether the cross does in fact mean a tick for this respondent, and code appropriately.

UNSTRUCTURED AND SEMI-STRUCTURED SCHEDULES

It was seen above that the process of coding a structured schedule involved devising a 'coding rule' which enabled responses to be transformed into standardized numbers. Thus the response 'male/female' was transformed into 1/2 by the 'coding rule': 'male = 1; female = 2'. Coding an unstructured or semi-structured schedule follows exactly the same logical process, but because of the variability in the format of the response the 'coding rules' must be that much more complex.

Let us look at a relatively straightforward example from a semistructured schedule and then a more complicated one from an unstructured schedule.

Semi-structured schedules

Dr John Pole has been conducting a survey of patient statisfaction with his services. He has persuaded his local Community Health Council to interview a random sample of his patients. One of the questions is an open-ended one:

How satisfied are you with Dr Pole as your GP?

The interviewers from the CHC wrote down verbatim the patient's replies. Here are a list of some of them:

A. He's an excellent doctor.
B. He can be a bit rude at times but he was spot on with George's arthritis.
C. I've never met him.
D. I always use the other partners.
E. He always comes when I call him out.
F. He's a terrible doctor... I always avoid him.
G. My diabetes has been a really worry ... and then there was Mary's cough ... drove me round the bend ... the medicine didn't work, though it's not his fault.
H. I get on with him though I know people who don't.

If Dr Pole had asked a closed question it might have been of this form:

Are you satisfied with your GP?   yes ☐
(Please tick)   no ☐
                                                             indifferent ☐

This could have been coded easily: 1, 2, or 3. We can try to use the same logic for the open-ended question, to score a similar 1, 2, or 3. The coding rule might be something like this:

Does the patient make positive comments?   Then = 1.
Does the patient make negative comments?   Then = 2.
Is it unclear whether comments are on balance
positive or negative?   Then = 3.

Using this schema, respondents A and E only have good things to say and would be scored 1. Respondent F is clearly negative and would score 2. Respondent B does make a passing negative comment but strongly qualifies it with a positive one. It would seem reasonable to score it 1. Respondent C has never met him so must be a 3. Respondent D's comment could be a negative one—perhaps he uses the other partners to avoid our doctor—but we can't be sure. A middle of the road '3' would probably be appropriate here. Respondent G goes on a bit but, while skirting close to criticizing the doctor ('the medicine didn't work'), denies the opportunity of making a critical remark. Certainly not a 2. Possibly that can be seen as a 'reluctantly' positive response and score a 1, or, being very cautious, a 3. Likewise respondent H gives two different opinions; but as we are interested in the respondent's own view it would seem right to score 1.

In this way the same sort of result as would be obtained from a closed question might result. Why therefore not use a closed question—it would be easier? Mainly because it is believed that the *quality* of the responses is better. Respondent B might have simply thought of the doctor's occasional rudeness and ticked the not satisfied box, whereas we might feel the actual view is more easily balanced, if not on the positive side. And so on. Taking this argument further means that if we can get more 'talk' from our respondents, the better the quality of our final scores.

In the example above we actually 'lost' data by classifying it into three boxes: we lost the ambivalence of B; we lost the diabetes and cough in G's account, and we lost the subtleties of the different ways in which patients arrived at an assessment of their doctors. Of course, in collapsing all those words into numbers we were bound to 'lose' data; however, the loss might not have been as great if our coding system had been more sophisticated. For example, in the coding we could have separated patient satisfaction with the GP's personal manner from satisfaction with his clinical competence, and gone through each statement in turn, making two separate scores (to be entered in two separate columns in the data-file). Thus respondent B would score a 2 on the interpersonal satisfaction scale yet a 1 on the clinical satisfaction scale; respondent H would score a 1 on the interpersonal and a 3 (for don't know/indifferent) on the clinical.

An alternative strategy for squeezing more and better-quality scores from the data would be to extend the satisfaction scales. Respondent A would seem to be far more glowing about the GP than H and yet with a dichotomous scale both would score a '1' for being satisfied. To encompass this we could code as under:

Strongly positive comments   = 1
Positive comments   = 2
Neither positive nor negative   = 3
Negative comments   = 4
Strongly negative comments   = 5

In this schema A would be a '1' and H a '2', while F would be a '5' and so on. If the data warranted it, the scale could be widened even further and/or other subscales created for different dimensions of satisfaction. Of course this process is limited by the quantity and quality of the 'talk data' collected. In this case only one comment was recorded for each respondent, but knowing what the coding scheme is, it would have been possible to guide the interviews to cover precisely these areas. Otherwise, if the coding system is too elaborate and the data are flimsy, we shall end up with most respondents in the 'unknown' category. However, the general principle is an important one and had the respondents been encouraged to talk more of their GP then more sophisticated coding frames would have been possible.

Remember that whereas coding frames for structured schedules can be devised *before* data is collected (because we know the limits of the answers), in the case of more open-ended questions we have to wait until we have seen the data before we can start to create appropriate frames. This latter task, of course, might more properly be done on data collected in a pilot survey so that one is prepared when data from the main study comes rolling in.

Unstructured schedules

The general principle of using some 'rules' to convert qualitative data into quantitative can be seen further in the analysis of masses of 'talk data', such as a tape-recorded interview using an unstructured or semi-structured questionnaire. Here we are able to look for much more subtle things than would be possible using structured techniques.

Dr Enid Hart believes that the worst cases of rheumatoid arthritis (RA) are found in women with poor self-esteem. (Wisely, she declines to put a causal inference on the observation as it could be in either direction: RA might cause loss of self-esteem just as low self-esteem might cause RA.) She decides to use the quantity of analgesics consumed as an indicator of the severity of the RA for the patient. To estimate self-esteem she interviews the women and tapes the conversation: she asks each about their lives and feelings of self-worth; the tapes last between one and two hours. Back in her study the pile of cassettes grows. The time has come to analyse them before other members of the family sabotage the study by replacing her data with Barry Manilow. Trapped amongst all the words recorded on the tapes is the respondents' self-esteem. How can it be extracted?

Rating scales

First Dr Hart must decide precisely what she is looking for. What is self-esteem exactly? If she doesn't know what it is, she is hardly likely to find it. Thus the task is both to define self-esteem and, from the definition, construct a *rating scale* which will act as a sort of template for scoring her patients. (In effect she is taking a 'concept' and operationalizing it; see Chapter 3.)

After much discussion with friends, and reading and thinking, Dr Hart decides that there are probably three components to self-esteem, namely:

(a)   feelings of value about one's body;

(b)   feelings of worth about one's mind/personality;

(c)   perceived quality of relationships with others.

Each of these components will need teasing out. Furthermore each component will need scoring on a scale. The length of this scale will depend on both the richness of the concept, i.e. her ability to distinguish different degrees of self-worth, and the richness of the data on cassette tape, i.e. will they be subtle enough to enable assignment to one of the points on the scale, or indeed to the scale itself?

Dr Hart discusses 'feelings of value about one's own body' with her colleagues. They agree that there must be a point at either end of the scale to represent either extreme pride and contentment in physical appearance or the absolute opposite. In between is more difficult. One of the colleagues points that that his feelings of worth vary—if he is well dressed he feels good; the other colleague says he feels awful after getting up and is glad there is no one there to see him. Dr Hart is beginning to get some points for her rating scale.

Always feeling one's body looks good	= 1
Some ambivalence about features of one's body but a feeling that these can be overcome with cosmetics, clothes, a good tan, etc.	= 2
Constant concern about some aspects of one's body, though relatively minor	= 3
More serious concern about one's body, of sufficient severity to affect interaction	= 4
Periodic bouts of feeling that one's body is ugly	= 5
Always feels that one is unattractive	= 6

It is important that Dr Hart's colleagues have helped devise this 'rating scale' because she will need them to help her by being 'raters'. It is obvious that raters must be very familiar with the scale they are using if they are all to use it consistently. Had Dr Hart devised the scale entirely on her own she would have had to 'teach' it to her colleagues and then ensure that they all had the same ideas by testing it on some pilot data.

Question 6(2)

Having devised the above rating scale on body perception Dr Hart wants to try it out. As one of her raters, how would you score the following transcripts taken from interviews recorded on a tape cassette. (Ideally you would listen to the tape itself in case tone of voice, pauses, etc. helped you in your ratings.)

W: Since I was a little girl I have known I had a weight problem ... it's just that nothing seems to fit ... it's probably because I like my food so much ... I find it so difficult to cut down ... the children don't help, they're constantly wanting cakes and things ... mind you, I'm getting to the point when it's hardly worth bothering with ... at my age, you know ... the only thing I worry about is diabetes ... my mother had it and they say it was her weight that did it, she was a big woman.

X: You wouldn't believe it now but I won a beauty contest when I was 17 ... and in those days it was all natural, not paint and purple hair like the young people today ... my husband said that my hair was my best feature, it used to be very long, but its just inconvenient to have it like that now, always getting in the way. My daughter's got long hair but she is young ... it's really lovely on her.

Y: I've been told that I've got a lop-sided face (laughs) ... but I can't be perfect all over ... size of nose indicates character I say ... besides its never done me any harm ... I've got a wonderful family and job so I leave the looks to those who are not so fortunate ... anyway a smile gets you through any day.

Z: I never let my husband see me without make-up on, I look dreadful ... first thing in the morning its a real struggle ... its difficult to hide puffy eyes and wrinkles, but by mid-morning I start to come alive ... some people are best in the morning, some in the evening, I always say and I am an evening person ... I suppose that if I went to bed early enough I wouldn't be so bad in the morning but then I'd miss the time I like the best.

These brief excerpts from the interviews have already been scored by three raters:

	W	X	Y	Z
Rater 1	4	2	2	4
Rater 2	3	1	2	3
Rater 3	3	2	2	4
Rater 4				

Add your scores to the table as rater 4. You will note that all the scores are not exactly the same for each respondent, but they are all similar, so it suggests that we are picking out something consistently from the interviews.

Because we have each been 'trained' to apply the same rating scale we can assume that we are, in effect, applying the same measure as each of us reaches our score. Going back to Chapter 3 on measuring things you will recall that the consistency of our scores is therefore a measure of the reliability of our test, in this case the application of our rating scale. In fact this characteristic of our rating scale has a special name, *inter-rater reliability*, and a special statistic associated with it (kappa) which gives a figure of 0 to 1: the closer the figure is to 1 then the more reliable our application of the rating scale. With appropriate training of raters it should be possible to achieve figures of 0.8 or 0.9 for inter-rater reliability.

Thus, by means of rating scales Dr Hart can extract from fairly dense qualitative data the exact numbers which will be entered in her data-file. She has followed the same process as if coding a structured schedule but in this case the 'rules' for assignment of cases are embedded in the rating scale and in the agreement as to how it will be used. But while the logic is not dissimilar, the use of rating scales has certain advantages and disadvantages over more traditional 'structured techniques'.

Advantages   1.   In principle the quality of the data we shall obtain will be that much better. A structured schedule relies on one assessor, the researcher or very often patients/respondents themselves, and offers a very narrow range of options. How is one expected to answer complex questions about feeling states—such as 'Are you happy?' in terms of 'yes/no' or 'a lot/a little' boxes? You might be happy with your job but find your golf handicap extremely worrying. Far better surely to capture an hour or so of someone talking about their life and basing rating scores on this comprehensive account. If well carried out, this latter process must surely produce a more valid measure.

2.   Structured schedules pre-categorize the data—a tick in a box—and if your questionnaire omitted a question it is forever lost. With unstructured data there is more flexibility, allowing a return to the collected data to derive even more measures. Of course there is a limit to this. An in-depth interview to explore life events and mood is unlikely to be of great value in assessing eating habits, but within those constraints there may be hundreds of measures that can be derived on a couple of hours of taped interview. For example, it may be that in our assessment of self-esteem we begin to realize that it might be the quality of the relationship with her husband which is the chief determinant of a woman's own feelings of self-worth; in which case we can create a rating scale for the quality of the relationship and go back to the interviews and apply it.

Disadvantages   The main disadvantage of devising rating scales to transform qualitative data into quantitative, as compared with coding structured schedules, is cost. Interviews require interviewers and, to get worthwhile material, may last several hours. The first ten minutes of any interview are likely to be fairly stilted, perhaps skirting around basic landmarks such as age, number of children, past illnesses, etc. But if the respondents are allowed the space to open up, then their more private selves are likely to emerge as the minutes tick by. On top of the time taken to conduct the interviews is the time to devise rating scales and the time to listen again to the tapes and apply the scales. Data quality might be good, but in the time it takes to process a dozen cases you might have collected and coded data from several hundred structured questionnaires.

In sum, it is swings and roundabouts. You can have large amounts of rather crude data or small amounts of more sophisticated. Which course you choose will depend very much on what your question is. Some questions are easily answered by structured questionnaires, others require the more time-consuming but finer techniques of collecting qualitative data and carefully transforming them into numbers.

QUALITATIVE METHOD

The final part of this chapter has shown how qualitative data can be transformed into numbers. The process is similar to that for obtaining numbers from quantitative data, in that 'categories' are imposed on raw data. Arguably, the use of rating scales, as suggested above, minimizes the 'loss' of detail in the data. Even so, there is still a considerable loss, and for some research the reduction of rich qualitative data to a few numbers would seem absurd. The alternative course of action is therefore to omit this transformation into number stage entirely.

Numbers obtained from coding frames and rating scales are 'manipulated', usually with statistical methods, to reach a general statement about the world, such as 'Only 60% of Dr Pole's patients are satisfied with his services' or 'Rheumatoid arthritics tend to have low self-esteem'. The alternative is to aim for this general statement direct from the data: there is still 'loss' of detail, but instead of abstracting numbers from the data, one takes more general 'themes' and uses these as the basis of the final statement. This 'manipulation' of number and themes will be further explored in the next two chapters.

SUMMARY

This chapter has dealt with the fairly technical procedure of transforming raw data into numbers. In addition it should, on reflection, enable you to see questionnaire design and interviewing in their context: if this is the point you have to get to, then your data collection should be so organized to enable you to get here.

SUGGESTED TASKS

1.   Devise a coding frame for the therapeutic groups of your prescriptions.

Take a sample of repeat prescriptions from your practice and code them using the above frame.

In addition, you may like to see if certain types of patients tend to receive more prescriptions from certain therapeutic groups than others. Note something of the personal characteristics of the patients receiving repeat prescriptions, code these, and compare them with your therapeutic groups. Are men more likely to get certain types of medicines compared with women? Are younger people more likely to get different types than older people?

2.   Using some case notes from the practice, devise a rating scale for the quality of information and legibility. Then take a random sample of case notes and, looking at the last five entries, code each using your prepared rating scale.

Are there any patterns? Do some doctors write fuller and more legible notes than others? Is it the type of illness or the type of patient that determines how good the notes are?

7 Analysing data

The previous chapter described how data was prepared and organized ready for the next phase, its analysis. Data comes through to this stage in different forms: it might range from being fairly 'raw', perhaps in the form of qualitative data such as taped interviews or conversation transcripts, to very 'refined' in the form of a string of numbers representing the coding of responses to a questionnaire.

The analysis provides the opportunity to link the research question (from Chapter 1) directly to the data which has been collected and 'organized' (Chapter 6). The exact form of the analysis will depend on the type and quality of data. If we have quantitative data, the chances are that we shall eventually move on to statistical tests (which are discussed in Chapter 8). But there are steps to cover before we get to this stage. These steps, which are covered in this chapter, try to show the logic of analysis. In practice you will probably find that you do not use all of them in any one piece of research, but by going through these formal steps you should appreciate some of the basic procedures in analysing data.

WHAT SORT OF DATA DO I HAVE?

In the chapters so far we have tried to avoid technical terms unless we think it is important that you know them, but before discussing data analysis you must be familiar with three sets of ways of categorizing your data, each with its own terminology. This, if you like, is the basic grammar we shall use in the chapter, and you need to become familiar with it before progressing to the next chapters.

Am I dealing with cases, variables, or values?

These are the terms with distinct meanings which you must be able to distinguish.

Cases
These are the individual 'things', some aspect of which you measure in your research. They are most likely to be patients, but they could be households, cars, tumours, or events, etc., depending on the research question.

Variables
These are the characteristics of the cases which you measure. Patients have

height, weight, blood pressure, stress, etc., all of which are variables. Equally, households have members, cars have colours and different engines, tumours have types and sizes, and events might have seriousness and timing. For any case we rarely measure all the characteristics or variables it 'possesses', only those which have a bearing on the research question.

Note that, depending on our research question and design, the same phenomenon might be a case or a variable. For example, in an investigation of suicide attempts in a practice one might consider the patients as cases who do or do not make suicide attempts (the variable), perhaps so that the characteristics of people who make attempts can be explored. Alternatively the actual suicide attempts could be the cases which, in their turn, have characteristics (variables) associated with them, such as patients' names. If there are several instances of multiple attempts at suicide in the practice, the latter schema allows for each attempt to be fully described (whereas using patients as cases makes each attempt simply another characteristic of the patient).

Values

These are the 'scores' for each variable. A patient might be 1.6 m tall, weigh 73 kg, and have a blood pressure of 130 systolic, 80 diastolic and suffer from 1.3 units of stress on the Noddy Stress Scale. In the same way, blue is the value for a car's colour, benign the value for a tumour's type, and 1945 the value for the date the Second World War ended.

Exercise 7(1)

Are the following underlined terms cases, variables, or values?

(a)   The doctor checked Mrs Smith's <u>blood pressure</u> and found that it was increased.
(b)   The doctor checked <u>Mrs Smith</u>'s blood pressure and found it was increased.
(c)   The doctor checked <u>Mrs Smith</u>'s blood pressure and found it was <u>increased</u>.
(d)   <u>Big families</u> often have more illness.
(e)   He looked <u>anaemic</u>.
(f)   I checked his <u>haemoglobin</u>.
(g)   She has had three <u>heart attacks</u>.
(h)   She has had <u>three</u> heart attacks.
(i)   <u>She</u> has had three heart attacks.

Suggested answers are given at the end of the chapter.

Are the variables dependent or independent?

In any research it is usual to divide the main variables into two sorts, independent and dependent. In a causal model the former is the cause, the latter the effect. Thus in a trial of analgesics for rheumatic pain the independent variable is the analgesic while the pain is the dependent variable (both being characteristic/variables of the patient/case who receives the drug or experiences the pain). An independent variable is therefore the thing that produces a change in the dependent one. (You can remember it by recalling that the dependent variable is the one that 'depends' on the independent.)

In a study with many variables it is simply a question of sorting out, on theoretical grounds, what affects what. A study of the effect of analgesics on rheumatic pain might also measure patients' nausea: as it is assumed that this, too, is brought about by the analgesic then this variable is also a dependent one. On the other hand, if we also measure the patient's age, believing that this might have an effect on pain perception, then this is an independent variable.

As we shall see later, some variables are less clearly dependent or independent. If in the above study we were able to measure the placebo effect, then this might be said to be brought about by taking the analgesic—hence it is a dependent variable—or it might be evaluated for its effect, alongside the analgesic, on the patient's pain, and therefore be an independent variable.

What is the level of measurement of the values?

Quantitative studies produce masses of numbers: but there are numbers and numbers. We have to be aware of what the numbers mean.

Question 7(1)

It has been suggested that different religious groups have different haemoglobin levels. To test this you conduct haemoglobin screening on 100 of your patients and your partner does the same. The coding frame you both use for religion is as follows:

> Protestant = 1
> Jew   = 2
> Catholic   = 3
> Other   = 4

Your partner reports to you that using these scores the average haemoglobin for his patients is 12.7 mg % and his average 'religion score' is 1.3. You have a larger Catholic population so he wonders if your average haemoglobin is different. You calculate your average haemoglobin level as 11.2 mg % and your religion score as 2.6—exactly twice that obtained by your partner. 'I think it looks like the higher the religion score then the lower the haemoglobin', your partner declares. What is wrong with his conclusion?

Your partner has added together numbers which cannot be added together. Haemoglobin is measured in milligrams. We know that a milligram scale has an essential property, technically called *transitivity*. This means that one milligram is much the same as any other. Thus the 2 mg between 5 mg and 7 mg is exactly the same as that between 2000 mg and 2002 mg. It means that 6 mg is twice 3 mg, and 9 mg is three times 3 mg. The fact that the increments on a scale are each exactly the same in this way means we have what is called an *interval scale*. Weight, length, volume, etc. are interval scales.

Our 'religion scale' possessed none of these properties. The fact that Catholics were scored 3 and Protestants 1 was entirely fortuitous; it expresses no mathematical relationship but was simply a cypher or name: hence such scales are called *nominal scales*. Perhaps we could have coded the religions A, B, C, and D which would not have tempted us to add together to create an overall 'religion' score. We can, of course, add the haemoglobins (an interval ratio scale) within A, B, C, and D. Thus the correct procedure in the above study would have been to find the mean haemoglobin for each religious group (1, 2, 3, and 4) and see if they were the same, or, as our hypothesis suggested, differed.

The third 'level of measurement' you will come across is an *ordinal scale*. As the name implies, an ordinal scale assumes some kind of underlying order or hierarchy, such that we can say that 3 is greater than 2, which in its turn is greater than 1, but we cannot say whether 3 is three times greater than 1 nor that 2 is twice 1. Imagine a line of numbers in an interval scale in which we randomly pick out several by underlining them:

$$1 \ \underline{2} \ 3 \ 4 \ \underline{5} \ \underline{6} \ 7 \ 8 \ \underline{9} \ 10 \ 11 \ 12 \ \underline{13} \ \underline{14} \ 15$$

These numbers (2, 5, 6, 9, 13, 14) are parts of an interval scale (6 is three times 2), but we could transpose it into an ordinal scale by numbering the first number 1, the second 2, the third 3, etc. We then have the following scale (with the original numbers in parenthesis):

$$1(2), \ 2(5), \ 3(6), \ 4(9), \ 5(13), \ 6(14)$$

You can see now that although our new scale looks like an interval one—running from 1 to 6—the numbers do not have the same properties as those in an interval scale. Thus, in this ordinal scale we know that 2 is not twice 1 (in fact it is two and a half times). In other ordinal scales we usually don't know the size of the 'gap' between the numbers, all we can say is that 2 is larger than 1, and 3 is larger than 1 and 2, and so on, but this is quite a lot more than we can say about a nominal scale.

Take, for example, a study to examine prescribing practices amongst different doctors. We might want to compare house officers, registrars, and consultants. Coding each respectively 1, 2, and 3, it might be reasonably claimed that we have an ordinal scale. It certainly isn't interval: two house officers is not the exact equivalent of a registrar; but neither is it nominal because there is an order or hierarchy to the scale: a consultant is 'more' in the sense of experience or qualifications than a registrar, who in turn is 'more' than a house officer.

At this stage it might appear a bit like an academic game trying to decide the level of measurement you have employed, but knowing what level of measurement you have is important, as we shall see, both in understanding what your data means and in choosing an appropriate statistical test.

Exercise 7(2)

Examine the following questionnaire and assess whether each question uses nominal, ordinal, or interval scales (N, 0, or I).

Patient questionnaire
Please answer the following questions:
1. What is your age in years?   □□
2. Are you male or female?   male □
                                                                 female □
3. What is your occupation?   [   ]
    How long have your been registered with your GP?
                                                        0–5 years   □
                                                        6–10 years   □
                                                        11 or more years □
5. Would you describe your health as:
                                                        Very good □
                                                        Good   □
                                                        Poor   □
                                                        Very poor □
6. Have you ever forgotten to take your tablets
    for your high blood pressure?   yes □
                                                               no   □
7. Mark somewhere on the line below your level of
    satisfaction with your treatment.

Very satisfied   Middling   Very dissatisfied
    └──────────────────────────────────┴────────────────────────────────┘

Suggested answers are given at the end of the chapter.

DATA CHECKING

It goes without saying that your analysis depends in part on the accuracy of your data. The whole research process up until now has been designed to ensure that your data is 'valid', but on top of that you must ensure that there are no silly errors from miscoding and mispunching. This requires checking your coding and usually double-punching the data. There are, in addition, a couple of things you can do to start off with: these are in fact part of the analysis but which might throw up any errors which have been made earlier.

First you might want to check *frequencies*. This means, in simple terms, seeing how 'frequently' various values occur. Thus, if your study was to measure the smoking habits of your practice population, it is useful just to do simple additions. What is the frequency of smokers in your adult population? 40%? 50%? This is what you might expect from national studies; if it turns out that you have only 10% or as many as 90%, then before you go on you had better check the figures; either there is a mistake somewhere, or you have a very unusual population, or you might have discovered something of great interest.

Similarly, if your study involved measuring consultation rates, it would be useful to know the mean (average) for the practice, together with the range. The national average is around 3 or 4 per year. About 20% of the population do not consult in any one year (so a good proportion of 0s in your data) and some people consult quite frequently. But if you find someone who consulted 80 times last year, it probably bears checking out: it may be correct but it is more likely to be an error than would be figure of 4 consultations per year.

At the end of this process you should have a fair idea of what is in your data, and, in addition, from picking up 'out-lying' values you will have performed another check.

The second way in which you might be able to check your data is by looking for *internal consistency*. Are all your examples of gynaecological problems to be found in women? A miscoded man would stand out here. Are all the people for whom you have details of how many cigarettes they smoke also scored as smokers? It is possible that you failed to get details of numbers of cigarettes smoked from someone scored as a smoker, but if you find a 10-a-day patient is also coded as a non-smoker, then something is wrong somewhere.

At the end of this preliminary analysis you will have:

● completed another check on the data;
● some basic descriptive statistics of your data;
● even more familiarity with your data, which should stand you in good stead when exploring it further.

HANDLING NON-RESPONDERS

Virtually all data collection produces blanks: patients who refused, notes that were missing, data that was illegible, and so on. The first stage of an analysis is to look at this 'non-response'.

The question to be answered is: are the non-responders different from the responders? If they are not different, then we can make the assumption that had they responded (or had the notes not been lost, etc.) then they would have answered in a similar way to responders. The way to check this is, as we advised earlier, to collect whatever data is available on non-responders so they can be compared.

Say, in a survey of symptom experience, 30% of the sample refuse to complete the questionnaire. If you manage to collect at least the age and sex of each of these non-responders, then you can see if their age and sex distribution mirrors that of the responders. If it does, then you can assume that their symptom experience would be likely to mirror that of the sample too. Of course, the more data you can use to make comparisons between responders and non-responders then the more sure you can be that the two groups are not markedly different. With this caution you can then proceed to analyse the data you obtained from the responders.

But what if the non-responders are significantly different in some way? Does this jeopardize the whole research study? Well, it does mean that your conclusions must be that more tentative, though you may be able to allow for some of the bias. For example, if you were to find that the non-responders were similar to the responders except they tended to be older, then it would seem wise, when you come to analyse the responders, to pay particular attention to age as a variable. Thus if, for example, it was found that older people do report more symptoms, then it is possible to draw some conclusions for the whole sample: in the light of the relative excess of elderly in the 'missing' part of the sample it is likely that they would probably experience more symptoms overall than those who did respond.

TWO-VARIABLE TABLES

There are now lots of complex statistical techniques for analysing many variables at once. You may at some stage wish to master these techniques, but be warned that their appeal is often more apparent than real because of the difficulty of interpreting the result. Even after a virtuoso performance with 'multivariate' statistics, researchers often come back to the basic building blocks of analysis: the relationship between two or three variables. This is as far as this chapter will take you because we believe that these are the most useful analytic tools. Let us start with two variables.

Unless your study is a simple descriptive one, e.g. how many asthmatics consult every year, you will have measured two or more variables in each of your cases. Let us imagine that you are interested in whether your female patients consult more frequently than male patients. You have some cases: these are your patients. For each case you measure two variables: sex and number of consultations per year. For each variable in each case you have a value: male or female and a number between, say, 0 and 10.

We can now draw up a 'table' which would look like this:

		Consultations during the year										
		0	1	2	3	4	5	6	7	8	9	10
Sex	male											
	female											

We can then assign each case to a 'cell' in the table. If the first case in the sample, a Mr Aaron, did not consult in the year under consideration, then he goes into the top left cell; the second case, Mrs Bell, who consulted three times, would go into the bottom row, fourth cell along; and so on. The result might be something like this:

Table 7.1.

		Consultations during the year										
		0	1	2	3	4	5	6	7	8	9	10
Sex	male	10	16	20	10	6	3	0	0	1	0	0
	female	2	1	4	3	1	2	1	0	0	0	1

This is a rather cumbersome table, having 20 cells many of which are empty. It can therefore be helpful to 'collapse down' the stretched-out 'interval' scale into a shorter ordinal one. Let's divide the group between 'high' consulters, having four or more consultations per year, and 'low' consulters, having three or less. The table can be redrawn:

Table 7.2.

		Consulters		
		low	high	Totals
Sex	male	56	10	66
	female	10	5	15

At first sight it would appear from this data that men are over two times more likely to be high consulters than women (10 versus 5 cases, respectively). However, this conclusion is mistaken because we are dealing with different sized groups of men and women—somehow the sample managed to include far more men than women (66 against 15). The question we are really asking is not 'What is the most likely gender of my next patient?'—which, from these figures would be male—but 'Comparing any individual man or woman, who is more likely to be a high consulter?' The way to answer this question is to express the results as percentages.

Thus:

Table 7.3.

		Consulters		
		Low	High	Total
Sex	male	85	15	100%
	female	67	33	100%

It now looks fairly clear that women tend to be higher consulters than men: one-third of women are high consulters in this table, compared with only 15% of men. We could explore this further by doing relevant statistical tests on either this table (or the first full one, Table 7.1) to see whether this distribution of consultation rates might have occurred by chance.

A note on percentaging

In Table 7.3 we percentaged across the row, ensuring that the figure 100% embraced either all the men or all the women. We could of course also have percentaged down the columns, making the 100% figure cover either low or high consulters. Deriving such a table from the original numbers in Table 7.2 we get:

Table 7.4.

		Consulters	
		Low	High
Sex	male	85	67
	female	15	33
	Total	100%	100%

From this table we might be inclined to draw the opposite conclusion than from Table 7.3: whereas in that table women seemed to be twice as likely to be high consulters as men, in this table—based on exactly the same data—it is the men who seem to be twice as likely to be high consulters than women. Which interpretation is correct?

In terms of the original question, Table 7.3 is correct. It is possible to use Table 7.4 but it answers a different sort of question. Usually the rule to follow is to make the independent variable total 100% in the table's margins because we are looking for the effect of the independent variable on the dependent one, in this case the effect of gender on consultation rates.

Papers do get published in which the researchers have percentaged in the wrong direction, so be on the look out for this mistake. Incidentally it makes no difference whether you put the independent variable along the top or down the side of the table so long as you percentage in the right direction (down or across respectively).

THREE-VARIABLE ANALYSIS

For simple questions analysis can stop at the two-variable stage. But the apparent relationship—or lack of one—between two variables can be further explored by adding in a third.

The logic behind this is simple. If we have two variables, X and Y, to which we assign values—present or absent—we can construct a two-by two table as we did above for gender and consultation rates:

Table 7.5.

		Y	
		present	absent
X	present		
	absent		

It is possible, though very unlikely in any research you will undertake, to have data which shows a perfect relationship between X and Y, such than when X is present Y is present and when X is absent Y is absent. For example:

Table 7.6.

		Y		
		present	absent	Total
X	present	100	0	100%
	absent	0	100	100%

It is much more likely to have relationships which suggest that Y is *partly* explained by X. For example:

Table 7.7.

		Y		
		present	absent	Total
X	present	80	20	100%
	absent	27	73	100%

What Table 7.7 means is that X certainly has an effect on Y, in fact quite a strong one, but change in Y is also being affected by some other factors; what causes Y to be present in the absence of X (top right-hand corner) and why does X have no effect on Y in over a quarter of all instances (bottom left-hand corner)? It is virtually impossible that your research is going to identify all the factors which affect Y such that change in Y is perfectly explained, but you can get further than Table 7.7 by introducing other variables which might influence Y, and look for their effect.

Specification

The process of examining the effect of introducing a third variable on an existing relationship between two variables is often called *elaboration* or *specification*, because we are trying to elaborate or specify the form of the relationship between our first two variables. Once you start you will see that there are many ways a third variable might affect another two. Here we shall go through two hypothetical examples to give a flavour of what can be found.

Example 1: the case of the iatrogenic clinic

For several years a practice ran a health promotion clinic for interested patients. It was then decided to evaluate the service and those men who had attended the clinic were compared with a control group of men of similar background who had not attended. By examining the notes, all myocardial infarctions (MI) in both groups were recorded. The partners were horrified to discover that the highest rate of infarcts (in fact twice as many) was in the group who had attended the clinic (Table 7.8).

Table 7.8

		Attenders	Control
MI	yes	5	2
	no	95	98
Total		100%	100%

The original hypothesis, that attendance at the clinic would benefit the patients, seemed to have been challenged.

However there are other possible explanations for this finding: the most promising is to argue that people who attended the clinic were more likely to be at risk in the first place, either through a poor family history or early signs of ischaemic heart disease (IHD), and this had induced them to try the clinic. Fortunately the GPs had recorded the patients' previous histories so it was possible to introduce these as a third variable into the analysis. In Table 7.9 only those men with any previous history of heart problems are included; in Table 7.10 only those without such a history. In effect we are 'controlling out' the effect of previous history. From these tables it is possible to see that the clinic, in fact, was not doing damage. Rather than the apparent model.

Clinic attendance → IHD

it seemed that the better model was:

Previous history → IHD
  ↘ Clinic attendance

in which a history of heart disease caused both attendance and the increased likelihood of an actual infarct.

Table 7.9. *Patients with a history of heart disease*

	Attenders	Control
MI yes	5 (9%)	1 (10%)
no	55 (91%)	9 (90%)
Total	60 (100%)	10 (100%)

Table 7.10. *Patients without a history of heart disease*

	Attenders	Control
MI yes	0 (0%)	1 (1%)
no	40 (100%)	89 (99%)
Total	40 (100%)	90 (100%)

Example 2: the case of the negative result

Concerned that unemployment might be causing ill health, a GP recorded the consultation rate of 100 of her patients who were unemployed and 100 employed patients to act as controls. She divided the consultation rates into two groups, low and high consulters. Placing the results into a table she found no difference between the two groups of patients:

Table 7.11.

		Employed	Unemployed
Consultations	high	15	15
	low	85	85
	Total	100%	100%

Perplexed at this finding, the GP decided to examine the relationship between employment and consulting, controlling for other factors. First she tried age, dividing the group into those under and those over forty (young/old). She obtained the following two tables:

Table 7.12.

		Young patients	
		employed	unemployed
Consultations	high	1 (2%)	12 (50%)
	low	59 (98%)	13 (50%)
	Total	60 (100%)	25 (100%)

Table 7.13.

		Old patients	
		employed	unemployed
Consultations	high	14 (35%)	3 (4%)
	low	26 (65%)	72 (96%)
	Total	40 (100%)	75 (100%)

From these it would appear that there was in fact a relationship between unemployment and consulting behaviour: for young men it increased but for older men it was diminished. The original table (7.11) had combined both and effectively cancelled out these two significant findings. It now would be interesting to go on and control for gender, as it might be hypothesized that men would react worse to unemployment than women; and then with other variables.

A NOTE ON PRESENTATION

Both the above examples used tables to present the data. After these have been put together they do need to be studied for a few minutes in order to decide what exactly they are showing. (The quickest way of seeing whether a two-by-two table contains anything of positive significance is to do a rough multiplication of the numbers at the end of the two diagonals: if they are roughly the same then the two variables in the table have little or no influence on each other; if, on the other hand, there is a large difference in the two sums obtained then there is a consequent large effect of one variable on the other.)

There are alternative to tables, and for early exploration of the data, graphs or histograms can be very useful. For example, when the dependent variable takes the form of an interval or ordinal scale as in the last example it is possible to get a visual comparison of the effect of two and three variables.

First let us see Table 7.11 plotted on a graph (but using the actual

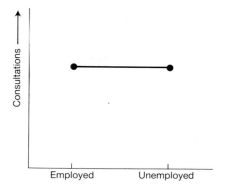

Fig. 7.1.   Diagram showing the relationship of employment to consultations.

consultation scale rather than the reduced two-value scale). The line in Fig. 7.1 shows the relationship between the two variables: it is flat because both employed and unemployed have the same 'rate' on the left-hand scale. Now introduce the third variable, age. This can be represented by two lines, one for younger and one for older men. It is now clear from Fig. 7.2 that for each age-group employment status does have an effect on consultations, as shown by the slope of the line; moreover, because the slopes are in opposite directions, we can conclude, as above, that the form of the relationship between employed and consultation varies inversely with age.

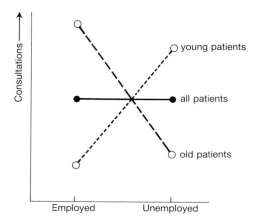

Fig. 7.2.   Diagram showing the relationship of employment and age to consultations.

MANIPULATING VARIABLES

We saw earlier how we could aggregate people of a certain age to form an age-group. In effect we 'collapsed' or reduced the possible values the variable 'age' could possess from a hundred or so to two (young/old) or at least many fewer (e.g. 0–9, 10–19, 20–29, etc.). In the same way we can manipulate our existing variables to create new ones. This is done by combining two or more variables to create a new one, usually because the new one has properties above and beyond those of the constituent variables. Let us look at three ways of creating new variables.

Rates

One of the most useful new variables to calculate is a rate. For example, if you have been comparing prescribing amongst the partners in your practice, you may have first measured how many prescriptions everyone wrote last week:

		Number of prescriptions
Doctor	A	80
	B	40
	C	50

Doctor A clearly wrote the most, fully twice as many as Doctor B. If you felt the practice was writing too many prescriptions, Doctor A would seem a good one to start on. Or would he? Another way of looking at the results is to calculate a rate which would express the number of prescriptions as a proportion of some relevant denominator. In this instance the denominator might be the number of patients seen last week (and then multiplied by 100 to get a prescription rate per 100 patients). This achieves the following result:

		Number of prescriptions	Number of patients	Rate per 100 patients
Doctor	A	80	160	50
	B	40	120	33
	C	50	90	56

The picture now looks quite different. The highest prescriber is not Doctor A but Doctor C.

There are, of course, other denominators which could have been used, such as personal list size, or the length of surgeries. In each case a choice must be made as to the most appropriate for the question in hand, but in each case this new variable can be used in the analyses in place of the 'raw' prescription numbers.

More complex combinations

In studies of risk factors, obesity may well be important. The commonest way of operationalizing obesity is by measuring weight. However, a weight which made one person obese might be normal in someone much taller. The solution has been to combine height and weight in a new variable using the formula:

$$\frac{\text{Weight}}{\text{Height}^2} = \text{Body mass index}$$

From starting with two variables we now have three: two have been combined (or reduced, as it is often described) into an index. We can, of course, go on to use all three variables in our further analyses, but it is much more common only to continue with the new one, which as we have seen is superior in certain ways to the old ones.

Indices

The logic of reducing variables to a summary index is a common one. In the above example it was achieved by multiplication and division, but it is often carried out simply by addition.

Say we were interested in patient satisfaction. We design a questionnaire to measure it, asking about satisfaction with the doctor's manner, competence, and facilities. If we scored each of these out of five, we could create a new 'general' variable of satisfaction by adding a patient's score on each of these 'subdimensions' of satisfaction, in effect producing a new index or scale running from 0 to 15, which can then be related to other variables that were measured.

This is the principle of index creation and is the basis of many measures in common use. An IQ score, for example, is a summation of different test items corrected for age; a personality test usually involves summing the results of a lot of different items; the General Health Questionnaire—a common psychiatric screening instrument—produces a single score by adding together questionnaire items. You can look at a diagnosis as a sort of index because various items (signs, symptoms, and investigations) have gone together to create a new overall summary category.

In Chapter 3 we discussed operationalizing concepts. For some, such as age, it was easy; for others, such as 'the quality of a relationship', it was more difficult, requiring a series of different questions to tap different components or dimensions of the concept. Now, at the analysis stage, is the point to put the components together again and to create the variable we were unable to measure directly.

A word of caution, however. Creating an index or new variable might seem like an easy task but there are difficulties that can make it very tricky. For example, taking the supposed three dimensions of patient satisfaction mentioned above: satisfaction with doctor's manner, competence, and facilities. If, as suggested, we simply add these, we make two important assumptions:

(1)   That the three five-point scales on which patients scored their satisfaction were in fact interval scales and not just ordinal (otherwise we could not legitimately add them together).

(2)   That each of the three 'dimensions' has equal importance or weight, otherwise we might have to 'weight' one or more of the scales (perhaps double the values of one which seemed 'doubly' important) in the calculation of the overall index.

In practice these two problems can make index construction a rather difficult business, especially when many variables are involved. There are some techniques available to help, but usually various assumptions have to be made. In terms of your own research, do try 'data reduction' by creating a new index out of small numbers of original variables, but remember to treat any results cautiously. New variables can be used in the analysis like the original ones, just as above.

QUALITATIVE DATA AND ANALYSIS

The 'rules' for analysing qualitative data are less precise than for quantitative. In quantitative data one is essentially looking for patterns between variables, using devices such as two- and three-variable tables to bring these to your attention. In qualitative data there is no such easy mechanism, although the same basic goal guides the analysis.

1.   Look for variables or themes

In qualitative research, as for quantitative, there are cases and for each case some data. But it is not clear at first what the variables are, because these emerge from the analysis. For example, in a study of patient satisfaction a questionnaire captures the researcher's views of what are important variables; the patient simply has to assign these variables particular values, e.g. a lot, not much, a little, etc. A qualitative approach to researching satisfaction, however, would perhaps invite patients to talk about how they saw satisfaction in general. The analysis then consists of looking at all the transcripts and drawing out the sorts of things that have concerned patients—which might be quite different from the ones the researcher imagined would have concerned patients. These patient-defined concerns are in effect the study variables.

2.   Identify more general statements of hypotheses which link variables

In the analysis of quantitative data it is usual to look at the values assigned to each variable of each case so as to explore the relationship between them. In a qualitative study it might not be necessary to go to the specific values before picking out a relationship between two or more variables. A patient who complains about surgery times because he works long hours allows us to generate the hypothesis that work patterns might affect patients' evaluations of surgery opening times. We might go on to other cases to see if a similar pattern emerges elsewhere. This process might be seen as equivalent to exploring the relationship between two variables in a table.

Then, akin to adding other variables, we would look for other patterns of relationships between work hours and surgery convenience: is it only men who complain about this? Is it evening and morning surgeries which are criticised? And so on. The end-result is a statement which somehow captures what is going on in the data.

QUANTITATIVE AND QUALITATIVE ANALYSIS COMPARED

It might appear that a quantitative demonstration of the relationship between working hours and practice facilities would be better than a qualitative one. Several points can be made in response:

1.   A quantitative study might not have measured these variables, not believing any of them to be important (though it would be possible to do so now that their importance has been suggested).
2.   A quantitative study tends to capture a response in a formal box; the respondent might give a more valid answer if allowed freely to express their ideas in their own words. The quality of data thus tends to be better.
3.   Sometimes 'patterns' in data which might be missed in a quantitative analysis can be more easily seen in qualitative data.

Taken together these points suggest that analysis of qualitative data, for all its seeming lack of precision, may produce important and interesting conclusions which would have been missed using more conventional techniques.

THE RESEARCH QUESTION IN THE CONTEXT OF THEORY

In Chapter 1 we stressed the importance of starting research with a question. That advice still stands, but we can now put it into a context. A research question ('What is the relationship between variable X and variable Y?') is not an isolated statement, but belongs to a group of lots of other statements about X and about Y. The single two-variable question is simply one component in a network of many interconnected variables which together make up 'theory'. For example, the statement that stress causes heart attacks is just one connection out of all the other factors which cause or influence in some way both heart attacks and stress.

In a rather simple way we started to build up a theory when we explored the relationship between attendance at a health promotion clinic, a history of heart disease, and myocardial infarction. Introducing more variables into that relationship would have allowed us to go on further in understanding the role of the factors involved.

The message from all this is that while our original research question might only involve two variables, it would be foolish just to measure and analyse those two variables alone. As we have seen above we might find no relationship between the two until we start to introduce other variables. Therefore in any research project it is important to try to tap and measure the other variables which might have an influence, even though they do not necessarily occur explicitly in the original research question.

How do you choose what to measure? In part this comes from the theoretical context of the question being asked. If you are carrying out a study of a supposed aetiological factor for ischaemic heart disease, then it would seem wise to include known risk factors, such as smoking, in the measurement process. Then there are some variables that from previous studies are seen to have very wide effects; it would be valuable to include them even though there might be no known connection between them and your question variables. Some socio-demographic variables (age, sex, social class, marital status, etc.) seem worth measuring in any study of your patients simply because they are so frequently found to relate to other patient variables.

On the other hand, in qualitative research what you look for is more guided by what you see and hear 'in the field'. Thus an observational study of a surgery waiting room will be dependent to a large extent on what actually happens there while it is being observed; or an interview with a patient on chronic illness will depend on what the patient has to say. Even so, you still need some guidance—what to look for, what prompts to give the patient—and these, too, will depend on having thought through the wider context of the research question in hand.

FINGERS, SLIDE RULES, AND COMPUTERS

Theory is important in another aspect of analysis. Nowadays most analysis is carried out by computer. The sorts of tables we constructed and discussed above can be called up almost instantly on a computer. Because of this there is a temptation to ask the computer for all possible tables in a sort of fishing trip for 'significant' results. This is not a panacea, however, for properly thinking through the meaning and interpretation of the data. If there are two variables, they can be expressed in one table; if we want to explore all the paired relationships between three variables, it will take three; four variables will take six; five will take ten; and so on. (This is not counting the tables generated by controlling for a third variable.) You can see that very rapidly you can get several hundred tables if you ask the computer to trawl every possible relationship. But, in addition to constructing the table, the computer can also give an instant evaluation of whether a particular relationship is statistically 'significant'. An advantage? Well yes, except that using standard 'levels' of significance, one in 20 tables will be reported as 'significant' simply by chance—and there is no way of discriminating these from 'really' significant results.

Use computers for analysis by all means, they are a great boon. There are now many statistical 'packages' available which will help you with the analyses outlined above; some of these packages work on personal computers so if you have a PC in the practice you might well be able to do the analysis on it. It will make the statistical tests covered in the next chapter very easy. (Ask at your local University Department of General Practice or Computer Centre for advice on what packages are available.) However, do not be seduced into believing that computers will do your thinking for you. It's your question, it's your data, do not let the computer take them over. The logic of analysis can be pursued quite independently of machines.

SUMMARY

This chapter has described the types of data you will have produced from your research project and the way to go about starting to analyse them using two- and three-variable tables. These tables will suggest interesting relationships between variables: but, you will need to ask the question, are they significant? This is a technical question which can be answered by use of appropriate statistical tests, which are discussed in the next chapter.

SUGGESTED TASKS

Monitor one week's surgeries, noting the age of each patient and whether they get a prescription or not. Draw up 2×2 tables to show the results. You would do this by splitting the ages into two groups; look at the effects of splitting at different ages, e.g. greater or less than 40, greater or less than 65, etc.

ANSWERS TO EXERCISES

Exercise 7(1)

(a)   Blood pressure = variable.

(b)   Mrs Smith = case.

(c)   Increased = value.

(d)   Big families = cases.

(e)   Anaemic = value.

(f)   Haemoglobin = variable (of which anaemia is a value).

(g)   Heart attacks = either case or variable depending on study design: is it patients or heart attacks which are being studied?

(h)   Three = value (of heart attacks).

(i)   She = case

Exercise 7(2)

1.   Age = interval ratio scale.

2.   Sex = nominal scale.

3.   Occupation = nominal scale—although if it were transformed into social class, it would become an ordinal one.

4.   Time registered = interval ratio scale.

5.   Health = ordinal scale.

6.   Compliance = nominal scale.

7.   Satisfaction = ordinal scale. (A visual analogue scale such as this might appear to be like an interval scale because exact gaps between responses can be measured. However, it is known that respondents are more inclined to mark a point towards the centre and ignore the extremes: this suggests that every millimetre of the scale does not have the same meaning for the respondent.)

8 Using statistics

'Don't be a novelist—be a statistician, much more scope for the imagination'
Mel Calman

The initial exploration of the data will produce some ideas about interesting relationships, some very clear, others suggestive. The task now is to determine whether the relationships between variables are as significant in the statistical sense as they seem to be when they are 'eyeballed'. In other words, those excess prescriptions given to adolescents may turn out to have no more importance than a chance variation, whereas the apparent small difference between prescribing rates to male and female elderly may turn out to be an important and 'real' difference.

How then should you set about examining the relationships between variables in a critical way so that the apparent will be separated from the real? The answer's easy—ask a statistician!

But just in case you don't have your own personal member of this quixotic species at hand, we will try in this chapter to explain the role of statistics in research. Statistics often frightens people: it can seem very complicated and mathematical. But don't be put off, the logic of statistics is a lot easier than the complex formulae and sums (which machines do for you these days anyway). We advise you to read this chapter through quickly at first. The best time to learn about statistics is when you have some of your own data and a question to answer.

In this chapter we shall try to give you an overview of where statistics fits in the research process by taking you through some of the basic tests used, employing as little mathematical skill as possible. At the end of the chapter you will:

- have some idea of which test to use in your individual specific circumstances;
- have some idea of when to use certain tests in general.

This hopefully will be a true 'Duffer's Guide to Statistics'.

Generally speaking, there are two main ways by which a knowledge of statistics can help to organize, sort through, and manipulate data which have been collected. First, some way is needed of *describing* the data. The mass of facts and figures should allow many things to be said about the sample looked at, but in its present form the data can probably be used to say very little. *Descriptive statistics* gives a variety of ways of presenting and summarizing the information collected so that it is intelligible to a third party.

However, research is about asking and trying to answer questions. Very often data has only been collected from a sample from a population in order to infer from the findings to that population. The second branch of statistics, *inductive* or *inferential* statistics, can be used to look at some of these areas. It is based on probability theory and allows estimates to be made from existing data of how likely the findings are to relate to the population from which the sample was drawn, or how likely it is that any hypothesis has been disproved. It uses more sophisticated, not to say at times convoluted, mathematical reasoning, but is a vital tool in research. We will return to some of the more simple aspects of it later.

So let's first of all look at various ways of organizing and presenting data. Let us start with an example which we shall use throughout the chapter.

NORMAN'S PROJECT

Dr Norman Curve, late of Puddletown Health Centre, now ensconced among the rolling hills of a single-handed rural practice, has decided to screen a sample of 35–40-year-olds for risk factors commonly associated with coronary artery disease. He wants to know how common are these 'common' risk factors, and whether they are associated with any other characteristics of the individual. Before embarking on a full screening programme for this age-range, he is particularly interested in knowing whether it will be worth screening both male and female populations. He therefore takes a random sample of 50 men and 50 women patients and invites them for screening. He decides to measure the following variables:

Concept	*Indicator*
Socio-economic status	Social class of main wage earner in household
Amount of exercise	Self-report (1–4)
Smoking	Self-report: yes/no
Blood pressure	Systolic BP
Amount of stress	Self-report (1–4)
Overweight	Body Mass Index (BMI)

The results from his sample are shown in Table 8.1 (p. 140).

Question 8(1)

How should Dr Curve represent the data to illustrate comparisons between the men and women in the sample for:

(a)   Social class?
(b)   Systolic BP?
(c)   Amount of exercise taken?

(a) *Social class*. Dr Curve needs to introduce some sense of order into the apparent chaos of his raw data. The first task therefore is to compile a *frequency distribution table*. He does this by compressing the data into summarizing categories. In the case of the social classification this would naturally fall into the five social classes (I–V), plus a group for the 'economically inactive' (EI) coded as '9'. This would produce Table 8.2.

Table 8.2.

	Social classes					
	I	II	III	IV	V	EI
Men	4	15	26	5	0	0
Women	3	13	29	3	0	2

To some extent, the way the information is categorized will depend on the *level of measurement* chosen for each variable (see Chapter 7). Is the data at the nominal, ordinal, or interval level of measurement? If it is interval, it is also necessary to know whether the scale of measurement is discrete, i.e. clearly defined differences such as number of children in a family, or whether it is continuously variable, as with height, weight, or BP. The number of categories chosen to summarize the data will therefore depend on the conciseness of the measurement, on the one hand, and the clarity of the proposed chart, on the other.

Perhaps a clearer way of representing the data given above would be by means of a *bar-chart*. In this the height of each bar represents the number in each group. (This is not to be confused with a *histogram* where the *area* enclosed by each rectangle is proportional to the frequency being illustrated.) When showing a comparison between groups, use can be made of shading or colour to distinguish between them.

(b) *Systolic BP*. Again, the first thing to do would be to construct a frequency distribution chart. From the raw data in Table 8.1, it appears that the measurement was done to the nearest 5 mm of mercury, so that initially this could be taken as the class interval, producing Table 8.3. A bar-chart could then be used to illustrate the findings between the two samples (Fig. 8.1).

Table 8.3.

	Systolic BP											
	110	115	120	125	130	135	140	145	150	155	160	165
Men	5	1	17	6	10	2	3	2	3	0	1	0
Women	0	3	1	20	7	9	1	7	1	0	1	0

Table 8.1. *Data set*

	Men						Women				
Social class	Exercise (0–4)	Smoking	Systolic BP	Stress (1–4)	Weight BMI	Social class	Exercise (0–4)	Smoking	Systolic BP	Stress (1–4)	Weight bMI
3	1	N	120	2	23	2	3	Y	120	1	20
2	3	N	120	1	20	3	0	N	130	2	26
2	1	Y	120	1	23	3	2	N	125	3	19
3	4	N	110	1	25	9	1	Y	120	1	27
3	2	N	120	2	23	3	1	Y	130	2	19
3	3	N	120	2	31	3	1	N	120	3	31
3	0	N	140	4	25	3	2	N	130	2	20
3	0	N	130	1	23	3	0	N	115	2	19
2	3	N	140	3	24	2	1	N	130	2	18
2	0	N	120	1	25	2	0	N	125	2	24
1	0	Y	130	1	29	3	1	Y	120	2	22
3	0	Y	130	1	25	3	0	Y	110	3	20
4	3	Y	115	1	26	2	2	N	120	1	20
3	1	N	120	1	20	3	2	N	120	1	25
4	2	Y	110	2	26	2	0	N	130	2	22
3	0	Y	120	2	28	3	1	Y	120	2	34
3	0	N	135	3	24	3	2	N	120	1	20
3	3	N	120	3	23	1	2	N	110	1	23
3	3	N	125	1	20	3	3	N	120	1	25
2	3	Y	120	2	27	3	2	Y	120	1	25
3	0	Y	110	1	25	2	0	N	120	1	21
3	3	Y	120	1	25	9	1	Y	120	3	26
4	3	N	125	2	26						

1	1	N	135	1	25	3	3	N	130	3	19
1	1	N	130	2	24	4	0	Z	110	3	23
2	0	Z	130	2	25	3	2	Y	120	2	25
2	3	Z	130	1	23	3	0	Z	125	3	22
3	0	Z	125	2	22	3	3	Z	120	2	21
4	3	Z	130	4	30	2	1	Z	155	2	26
3	2	Y	120	1	25	3	3	Y	120	1	27
3	0	Z	160	2	24	1	1	Y	120	2	18
2	0	Y	130	1	21	3	3	Y	125	2	23
3	0	Y	145	3	28	3	3	Z	140	2	21
2	0	Z	150	1	22	2	0	Z	120	1	23
2	2	Y	150	2	23	2	0	Z	140	2	21
3	3	Z	140	3	25	3	2	Y	125	2	20
2	0	Z	150	2	24	4	1	Y	140	2	21
1	4	Y	120	2	25	3	0	Z	125	1	26
3	0	Z	125	2	26	2	0	Y	120	2	24
3	2	Y	130	1	25	1	2	Y	140	2	21
3	0	Y	130	2	25	3	2	Y	135	2	25
3	2	Y	110	1	29	4	0	Z	145	3	29
2	0	Z	125	1	20	3	0	Z	140	1	28
3	1	Y	125	1	27	2	2	Z	130	1	23
4	2	Z	120	1	25	3	3	Z	120	2	23
2	1	Z	110	1	23	3	2	Y	130	1	21
3	0	Z	120	2	25	3	0	Y	140	2	21
2	3	Y	120	1	24	3	3	N	120	1	27
2	0	Z	120	1	21	2	1		130	1	22
3	2	Y	145	1	26		3		140	2	21

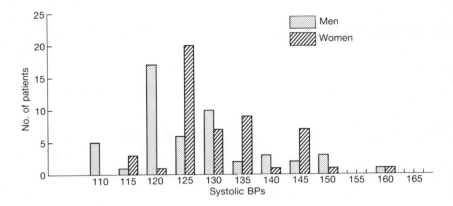

Fig. 8.1.   Bar chart of systolic blood pressures.

An alternative method of demonstrating the data might be to produce a cumulative frequency curve, also known as an *ogive* (Fig. 8.2). In this, the number in each group is added, going up the range. In our example the number of men with a systolic BP of 110 would still be 5, but for 115 would be 1 plus the 5 already counted, and for 120 would be 17 + 1 + 5, and so on. Demonstrating the data in this way makes it easier to answer questions such as 'How many of the sample had systolic pressures below 130?', or 'At what systolic BP were half the sample above and half below the figure?'.

(c)   *The amount of exercise.* As before, the first task to complete is to construct a frequency distribution table (Table 8.4). Here there are only five categories, and it may be that the clearest way of demonstrating the

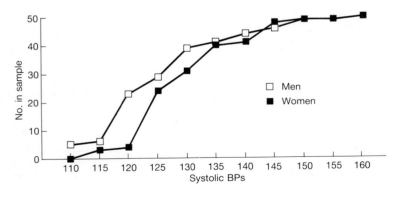

Fig. 8.2.   Cumulative frequency curve of blood pressures.

Table 8.4.

	Amount of exercise taken				
	0	1	2	3	4
Men	20	7	8	13	2
Women	15	11	14	10	0

data is with a couple of *pie-charts*—circles divided into sectors, one for each value of the variable. The area of each sector represents the proportion of the sample having that particular value. These are particularly easy to construct using commonly available graphics packages for personal computers.

In the present example, there are five possible values, 0–4, for the amount of exercise taken. Two circles are needed, one for the sample of men, and another for the women, and each would be divided into five sectors. The size of each sector is calculated using simple arithmetic. The whole sample comprises 50 cases—therefore the complete circle represents 50 cases. There are 360 degrees in a circle, and so in this example one case would be depicted by 360/50 degrees. Each sector size can thus be found by multiplying the number of cases with that particular value by the proportion of the circle representing one case. This is illustrated in Table 8.5. A pie-chart could now be drawn, together with the corresponding one for the sample of women (Fig. 8.3).

Table 8.5.

	Amount of exercise taken by the men				
	0	1	2	3	4
Number	20	7	8	13	2
Degrees	$\dfrac{360 \times 20}{50}$	$\dfrac{360 \times 7}{50}$	$\dfrac{360 \times 8}{50}$	$\dfrac{360 \times 13}{50}$	$\dfrac{360 \times 2}{50}$
=	144	50	58	94	14

So it is clear that there are various ways by which the data can be displayed to illustrate points or to highlight and suggest differences. The method chosen will depend on how the results have been classified, and especially on the number of categories into which the data have been placed.

Exercise 8(1)

Construct tables and charts to present and contrast the results from the two samples for:

(a)   smoking behaviour;

(b)   self-assessment of stress factor;
(c)   ideal weight distribution.

Suggested answers are given at the end of the chapter.

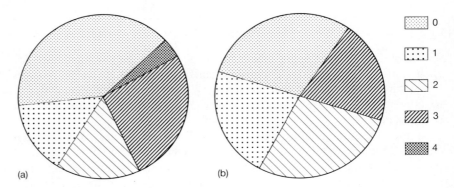

Fig. 8.3.   Pie-charts of exercise taken (a) by men and (b) by women

SUMMARIZING DATA

For many statistical tests one needs to develop a method of summarizing the values found for a variable—a kind of 'average' figure for all the data. There are two features about the data collected that are usually looked at in trying to summarize and describe the variable:

(1)   A measure of central tendency.

(2)   A measure of the degree of dispersion of the data.

To give a simple example: If you were one of four partners in a practice and you were asked to describe the age-structure of the partnership, but were only allowed to use one figure, then you might add all the ages up and divide by four—this would give the *mean* for the data. This 'average age' might be 41. However, although very concise, this figure may hide the fact that the ages of the partners are 27, 27, 28, and 83. A measure of the *dispersion* of the data might have given a third party a much clearer idea of the ages of the partners: 'My partners' ages vary from 27 to 83.'
    'Might as well give all the ages in that case.' You're right. Giving all the results gives the most information, and is just as easy to do with only four cases to report. But when it comes to the 50 cases in Norman Curves's samples, or the many thousands that might comprise a sample in a large research project, one sees the need for summarizing the data. And not only are these summarizing statistics occasionally more convenient, but they are very important since they often form the basis of many other statistical tests.

MEASURES OF CENTRAL TENDENCY

The arithmetic mean

As we have seen the mean, or average, is a commonly and easily derived figure. It is found by adding together all the values found for a given variable and dividing by the number of cases. So, in the data in Norman's screening project it is a straightforward task to calculate the mean systolic BPs for his male and female samples.

There were 50 observations for both samples. Adding the readings together for the men gives a total of 6345; which when divided by the 50 readings gives a mean systolic BP for the men in the sample of 126.9. Similarly the 50 systolic BPs in the women added together produces a total of 6305, and a mean systolic BP of 126.1.

Exercise 8(2)

Calculate the mean Body mass Indices (BMI) for both the male and female samples.
Suggested answers are given at the end of the chapter.

The mean is a widely understood and easily calculated figure, which takes into account all of the data within a group. However, as with the simple example of the partnership age-structure, a few items of a very high or low value may result in the mean being a misleading figure in representing the distribution of values within the group. For that reason, unless it seems fairly clear that the values are evenly and symmetrically distributed over a fairly narrow range, then it may be better to choose one of the other measures of central tendency.

The median

The median is defined as the middle item in a distribution, that is the figure for which half the cases have a value less and half more. Obviously, to calculate it, all the cases in the sample have to be arranged in numerical order. If there are an uneven number of values in a group, then the median is the middle number. For example, if the four partners took on a fifth partner, aged 56, the ages of the partners would now be:

27,   27,   28,   56,   83.

In this series the median age would be 28, because there are a equal number of values (2) both below and above it in the series. If there are an equal number of cases in the group, the median is conventionally taken as the mid-value between the middle two. Again, in our partnership example, if the practice took on a sixth partner, aged 35, the ages would now be:

$$27, \quad 27, \quad 28, \quad 35, \quad 56, \quad 83.$$

The ages of the middle two cases in the series are 28 and 35. Therefore in this series the median value would be the mid-point beween these two values, $(28 + 35)/2 = 31.5$.

Question 8(2)

In the screening project, what are the median values for the male and female samples for:

(a)   Amount of exercise undertaken?
(b)   Amount of stress felt?

Since the sample size is 50 the median value will, in all cases, lie between the 25th and 26th values. For the men, the amount of exercise taken by the 25th and 26th members of the sample when arranged in order is 1. Therefore the median figure for exercise in the male sample is $(1 + 1)/2 = 1$. In the female sample, again both the 25th and 26th figures equal 1, and the median is also 1.

In (b), the amount of stress felt by the 25th and 26th members of the male sample, when the figures are arranged in numerical order, is 1, and again the median is 1. For the female sample, both the 25th and 26th members of the series have a value of 2, and so in this case the median value for stress felt by the women in the sample is $(2 + 2)/2 = 2$.

Exercise 8(3)

Calculate the median values for both the male and female samples for:

(a)   systolic BP;
(b)   BMI.

How do these figures compare with their mean values? Can you make any suggestions as to why they should differ?

Suggested answers are at the end of the chapter.

There are two other values worth mentioning, which are derived in similar fashion to the median. These are the *quartiles*. As with the median, all the values for a variable in a series are ranked in order. The *upper quartile* represents that figure in the series which the top 25 per cent of the values in the series exceed, and the *lower quartile* has 25 per cent of the series with values less than it. Their relationship to the median can best be shown by using the cumulated frequency chart, discussed and demonstrated earlier, and as an example, the relevant chart for the systolic BP

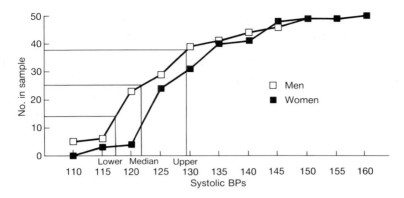

Fig. 8.4. Quartiles of blood pressure.

readings for men would show the quartiles and median as in Fig. 8.4. Note that the median is, in effect, the 50th percentile.

The mode

The mode again represents a type of 'average'. It is defined as the most frequently occurring value in a distribution, and the class with that value is called the *modal class*. A common use of it occurs when we talk about the 'average partnership having 3 partners in it' (even though the mean might actually be 3.124).

Question 8(3)

What is the modal class for the social class of Norman's two samples?

From the bar-charts derived earlier it can be seen clearly that the modal class for both samples was social class III, in which there were respectively 26 and 29 of the men and women in the samples.

SUMMARIZING DISPERSION

Measures of central tendency are limited to a greater or lesser extent in their ability to describe the distribution within a sample of the values for a measured variable. Therefore other figures are used to give some idea of the spread of results.

The range

This is the simplest way of describing a distribution. The range simply describes the spread from the lowest to the highest in the series. Therefore, back at our four-man partnership we could have said that 'the ages of the partners range from 27 to 83'. This certainly tells more than did any of the measures of central tendency, and if used in conjunction with one of those measures would allow a fair guess at the underlying distribution.

The inter-quartile range

However, as in the above example, one or two extreme results might cause mistaken assumptions to be made. To avoid this, use is occasionally made of the inter-quartile range, which, as the name suggests, is the range between the low quartile and the high quartile met earlier. This, in effect, excludes both the lowest and highest 25 per cent of results.

Question 8(4)

What are the ranges and inter-quartile ranges for both samples for:

(a)   systolic BPs?
(b)   BMIs?

For the men, the systolic BPs vary from 110 to 160, therefore the total range is 50. The inter-quartile range will lie between the 12th/13th readings and the 37th/38th. In the case of the men the readings are 120 and 130, thus the inter-quartile range is 10. For the females, all the readings range from 110 to 155, a total range of 45. The quartile figures are 120 and 130, and so, as with the men, the inter-quartile range is 10.

For the BMIs, the values for the men were from 21 to 31, a range of 11, and for the women from 18 to 34, a range of 16. The quartiles for the men were 23 and 26, an inter-quartile range of 3. The corresponding figures for the women were 20.5 and 25, with an inter-quartile range of 4.5.

These various ranges give some idea of the dispersion of data around the central point, but can still mask the true *shape* of the distribution of the results. These shapes can be of many forms, but there are a few common ones. In Fig. 8.5a, the distribution of the frequency of occurrence of the results adopts a symmetrical shape, clustered around the mid-point, and the mode, median, and mean all coincide. This bell shape, which is found with many interval-based biological data (such as height, weight, BP), is called the *normal* distribution.

Figures 8.5b and c are examples where the results have clustered towards one or other extreme. These are called *skewed* distributions, negatively in the case of (b), where the clustering is to the right of the mean, and positively in the case of (c), where it is to the left. Figure 8.5d is an example of another distribution occasionally met, where there are two peaks in the distribution of the results—this is a *bi-modal* distribution.

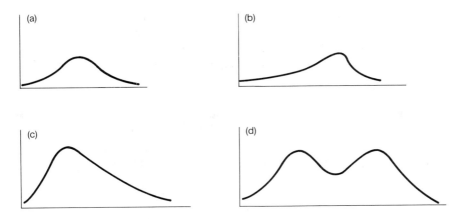

Fig. 8.5.   Distribution curves.

Obviously, none of the summarizing figures we have met so far will tell us anything about the underlying shape of the distribution curve.

The standard deviation

Because the range and inter-quartile range are limited in their application, the *standard deviation* is often employed to describe dispersion, although it can only be used in symmetrical and uni-modal distributions. It would be of limited value in either of the severely skewed distributions shown above, or with a bi-modal distribution.

The standard deviation gives an idea of the spread of results around the arithmetic mean and hence gives an idea of the height of the curve. The greater the dispersion and spread of results, the greater the relative standard deviation, and the flatter the curve.

It also has other important properties. If the shape of the distribution curve is normal, it is possible to show that 68 per cent of the results will fall within one standard deviation either side of the mean, and that 95% of the results will fall within about two standard deviations (actually 1.96) either side of the mean (Fig. 8.6).

Therefore, if we measured the heights of the next 100 adult male patients and found that the mean height of this sample was 5 ft 9 in, with a standard deviation of 2 inches, we could say (since we know that height is a normally distributed variable) that 68% of the adult males in the sample would have a height between 5 ft 7 in and 5 ft 11 in, and that 95% would between 5 ft 5 in and 6 ft 1 in.

The standard deviation is a measure of the dispersion of results around the mean and that is therefore exactly how it is calculated.

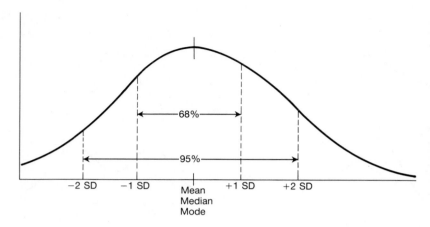

Fig. 8.6.   The normal curve—more detail.

- The mean of all the results in the sample is calculated.
- Each of the results is now taken in turn and the difference between it and the mean worked out.
- Some of the results will be greater than, and some less than the mean. This means that some of the differences will be greater (+) and some less than zero (−). To remove the negative values, all these differences are squared.
- These squared differences are added together.
- This sum is divided by the number of results.
- The square-root of this figure is now taken to give the *standard deviation*.

Let's look at an example. You have joined your new partnership of five with ages 30, 35, 45, 53, and 62. The mean age of the partners is 45. Laid out in a table we see:

Age	Mean age	Deviation	Squared deviation
30	45	−15	225
35	45	−10	100
45	45	0	0
53	45	+8	64
62	45	+17	289

For each case in the series the difference is calculated between its value for the variable under consideration (age), and the mean for that variable in the series. If we had simply added these deviations from the mean together, the effect of the signs (+ and −) would have been to cancel each other out. We could have simply ignored the signs and added the deviations and derived a *mean deviation*, in this case 50/5 = 10. The usual way is to square the deviation, in effect removing the sign.

If we now total these squared deviations it comes to 678. This total, divided by the 5 cases, gives a mean squared deviation of 135.6. This figure is also known as the *variance*. The standard deviation is found by taking the square root of this figure, which in this example is 11.6.

The shorthand, or formula, which describes this process of calculating the standard deviation is:

$$SD = \frac{\Sigma x^2}{n}$$

Where: SD represents the standard deviation; Σx^2 represents the sum of the squared deviations from the mean; and n is the number of items in the series.

Question 8(5)

Calculate the standard deviation for the systolic BPs in the male sample.

First compile a table based on the frequency table as follows:

Value	Mean	Deviation	Squared	No. with value	Total deviation
110	127	−17	289	5	1445
115	127	−12	144	1	144
120	127	− 7	49	17	2448
125	127	− 2	4	6	24
130	127	3	9	10	90
135	127	8	64	2	128
140	127	13	169	3	507
145	127	18	324	2	648
150	127	23	529	3	1587
160	127	33	1089	1	1089
				Total	8110

Number in group = 50;
Mean squared deviation = 162.2;
Standard deviation = $\sqrt{162.2}$ = 12.7.

If we were to assume that the results in our sample were normally distributed, we could now say that 68% of the results would fall within one standard deviation of the mean, that is in the range 127± 12.7, say 114 to 140. In fact 39 of our results do, that is 78%. Similarly we could predict that 95% of the results would fall in the ranger 127 ± 25.4. In fact 49, 98% of our results do.

Exercise 8(4)

Find the standard deviation for the BMIs for the two samples. Do you think they are normally distributed?

Suggested answers are at the end of the chapter.

MAKING DECISIONS—INFERENTIAL STATISTICS

So far we have concerned ourselves with looking at ways of presenting and summarizing our data. However, we pointed out at the beginning of this chapter that this is only one limited use of statistics. Often we want to use the data we have collected to make some decision or statement about the population from which the sample or samples have been taken. In drawing a random sample from a population—say a one in ten sample of the over-65s from the age–sex register—we hope that the sample will be typical of the whole population. But, of course, with some smallish samples chance biases can easily creep in. Yet the logic for the whole research is to be able to say something about the total population (i.e. all the over-65s in the practice), and not just the one in ten sample. Statistics can come to the rescue here. It will allow us to estimate how closely our sample findings are likely to be to the population's actual characteristics without actually having to go to the often impossible length of measuring the latter.

On the other hand, it may be that we are comparing measurements from two samples and we want to know whether any difference noted is a real difference or whether the difference is just a chance variation to be expected when drawing different samples from the same population.

Chance and probability

Underlying many statistical decisions is the attempt to decide how likely it is that any one result can have been expected to occur by chance. Thus the chance that I can guess your birthdate correctly would be one in 365, or 0.003. The probability that 'all men will die' is 100% or 1.0. Usually probabilities are expressed in relation to this standard of unity. If an event occurs by chance 1 in 10 times, it has a probability of 0.1, one in twenty 0.05, one in a hundred 0.01, one in a thousand 0.001, and so on.

In medical research it has conventionally been taken that if it is calculated that a given result would have occurred by chance only 1 in twenty times, $p = 0.05$, then it is more than likely that this is a 'real' finding and not a 'fluke' or chance result. For example, if a new hypotensive agent is found in a trial to reduce blood pressure by more than a placebo, it might be calculated that there was a 1 in 20 chance that such a result might be a random fluke. However, the convention is to ignore this latter possibility if the chance is 1 in 20 or greater, and accept that it is the drug that is working rather than chance. We say in this case that the result is 'statistically significant at the 0.05 level'. This attempt to quantify the likelihood that any given result or difference between results could have occurred by chance is all that most inferential statistical tests are about. At the end of the day they still make no absolute statements about the 'truth' or otherwise of your findings. An unusual result which your tests suggest would have only occurred by chance 1 in 20 times ($p = 0.05$) could still be that chance finding. Hopefully these issues will become clearer as we proceed through the remainder of this chapter.

The normal curve

We have spent some time in this chapter looking at some of the characteristics of the normal curve. Now you have seen it, what can you do with it?

The normal curve has one or two interesting characteristics, especially the fact that 68% of figures in a normally distributed sample will lie within one standard deviation of the mean, and that 95% will lie within two standard deviations of the mean. This can be used to make statements about an individual value in a sample, but more commonly we are interested in how our sample represents the population from which it was drawn.

The standard error of the mean

We briefly looked at the concept of the standard error in Chapter 2, when we used it to try to predict the size of sample we should be thinking about using when designing our project. You may remember that any one sample is unlikely to give the exact true mean of the population from which it was taken. If a large number of samples was taken, it would be found that the results for the means of all these samples would tend to cluster around the true mean of the population in a *normally distributed* pattern. The standard deviation of this distribution of these sample means is called the *standard error of the mean*. Therefore we know that 95% of all sample means from this one population will fall within two (or 1.96, to be precise) standard errors of the true mean. Using the result of the one sample usually available can allow a start in making assumptions about the underlying population with a known degree of mathematical certainty.

But hold on—how do you calculate the standard error of the mean for a population when you have only taken one sample? Surely you don't have to replicate your sampling exercise a dozen times?

Luckily it is possible to calculate the standard error from your one sample as long as you know:

(1) The mean of that variable in your sample.
(2) The number of cases in your sample.

(3)   The standard deviation for that variable in your sample.

Armed with these results there is a formula that allows a calculation of the standard error:

$$SE = \sqrt{\frac{SD}{n}}$$

where SD is the standard deviation for that variable and *n* is the number of cases in the sample.

It is clear from this that the size of the standard error will depend on the size of the sample, as was pointed out in Chapter 2.

Question 8(6)

From a sample of 50 males aged between 35 and 40 years old drawn from the practice (Table 8.1), Dr Norman Curve established that the mean systolic BP was 126.9. His practice list of 10 000 patients probably contains several hundred males in the 35–40 age-group. What statement could he now make about the systolic BP of all the males in the practice aged between 35 and 40?

He knows the following:

$$
\begin{array}{ll}
\text{Mean systolic BP} & = 126.9 \\
\text{Standard deviation} & = 11.4 \\
\text{Number in sample} & = 50
\end{array}
$$

Therefore, substituting into the equation above he can calculate the standard error of the mean:

$$SE = \sqrt{\frac{11.4}{50}}$$
$$= 1.6$$

As a result of the characteristics of the normal curve he knows that the sample result of 126.9 will, 19 times out of 20, lie within two SEs of the true mean systolic BP. In other words there is a 95% probability that the true mean systolic BP of all 35–40-year-old males in his practice will lie somewhere between 126.9 ± (2 × 1.6), that is between 123.7 and 130.1.

Since the standard error is inversely proportion to the sample size you may like to consider what he could have said about the true mean had the same results be obtained from larger samples of 100 and 200 patients.

With a sample of 100 the SE would have been 1.1, and so the true mean of that population of 35–40-year-old males was likely (19 times out of 20) to be in the range 124.7–129.1. A sample size of 200 producing the same results would have given a SE of 0.8, and so there would have been a 95% chance that the true mean was between 125.3 and 128.5. Another way of saying this is that at the 95% *confidence limits* the true mean lies between 125.3 and 128.5.

Exercise 8(5)

Calculate the standard errors for the BMIs for both the samples of males and females drawn from Norman's practice and displayed in Table 8.1.

What can you say about the BMI for males and females aged between 35 and 40 in his total practice population?

Answers are given at the end of the chapter.

COMPARING SAMPLES

When we compare two results to see if there is any difference or change, e.g. when investigating the questions: 'Does Skinnyfax cause weight loss over six months?', or 'Is depression more common among women compared with men?', what one does in fact is to compare the results that summarize the central tendency or distribution of the two sets of results. This is done to see whether any differences that are found between these two results could be explained by the element of chance inherent in any sampling exercise, and that, therefore, there is no real difference between them. Another way of expressing this is say that the object of the exercise is to see if the two samples were from the 'same' population. Thus, if people weigh the same both before and after Skinnyfax, they can be said to be from the same population, irrespective of whether they were drawn before or after the drug was given.

It is usual to assume in the first instance that any differences that are found between the two samples have arisen by chance, and this is the reason that hypotheses are stated as *null hypotheses*. The research hypothesis may be that 'Skinnyfax causes a loss in weight', but for the statistical test the opposing null hypothesis is stated: 'Skinnyfax does not cause a loss in weight'. In other words, any differences in weight loss found in the treated and untreated samples are purely to be expected by chance, and can be explained by the expected distribution of the means of such samples (given their size and the usual spread of the variable being measured). However, if the differences found suggest that such results would be likely to occur by chance on less than one in 20 occasions, then this suggests that the null hypothesis has not been supported. Therefore, the hypothesis that Skinnyfax does not cause weight loss would be rejected (and by implication the conclusion drawn that it does cause weight loss).

DIFFERENCES OR ASSOCIATIONS?

So far in this part of the chapter we have looked at samples and their relationship to the population from which they were taken. We have said that it is possible to make statements about how likely it is that two samples have come from the same population. For example, we can ask 'Are men more likely to be overweight than women?', and look to see whether there is evidence for a *difference* between the BMIs for the male and female samples. Do they appear to come from the same population or is there evidence that they are two samples from different populations? Do children who clean their teeth regularly have fewer caries than those who don't? Has drug X caused a fall in serum potassium?

However, often we are trying to suggest more than that. We may try to show that the more you have of X the more you are likely to have of Y. Here we are beginning to try to show an association or correlation between the variables. We are trying to make some statement about *how much* one variable is associated with or changes with another, e.g. height and weight, number of cigarettes smoked and the incidence of lung cancer, socio-economic status and health. Not only might there be a difference in the amount of health between the 'rich' and the 'poor', but data suggests that the less of 'richness' you possess, the less of 'health' you have. The correct statistical test has to be chosen to allow that much more to be said about the data.

There are a whole battery of statistical tests and probably even more thin, thick, and very thick textbooks written about them. You may feel the need after this brief introduction to rush out and buy one, but in the meantime we can offer some basic guidance about deciding which test to use.

One limiting factor on the precise test you can use will, in most cases, be the level of measurement of the variables being examined. Therefore the first step is to ask yourself: 'What level of measurement have I used for the variables I have?' We have already discussed, in the previous chapter, levels of measurement—nominal, ordinal, and interval. The lower the level of measurement, the more restricted are the number of tests that can be used.

If the data have been measured on an interval scale it is then possible, by looking at the frequency distribution curve for your data, to ask a supplementary question: 'Is the data normally distributed?' Then a useful way of proceeding is to devise a simple table to summarize your data, as in Table 8.6. For example, for the question 'Are men more overweight than women?', we could summarize the data as in Table 8.7. If we ask whether

Table 8.6.   *Data summary table*

Variable	Value	Level of measurement

Table 8.7. *Data summary table (weight and sex)*

Variable	Value	Level of measurement
weight	BMI	interval
sex	M/F	nominal

Table 8.8. *Data summary table (weight and blood pressure)*

Variable	Value	Level of measurement
weight	BMI	interval
blood pressure	systolic reading	interval

systolic BP increases with the degree of overweight, we might possibly end up with Table 8.8.

If the measurements are not at interval level, or if there is doubt as to whether or not they are normally distributed, then the tests that can be used are those suitable for *non-parametric* (i.e. non-normally distributed) data.

In some textbooks you will find aids to help in deciding which test to employ—usually in the form of a decision tree or table. Figure 8.7 is one such guide. We will briefly describe the commonly used tests later, but first of all try using the decision tree.

Question 8(7)

We have decided to see whether people who smoke have higher blood pressure than non-smokers. Our questionnaire asked the question, 'How many cigarettes do you smoke each day?', and the blood pressure of each person in the sample was measured in mm of mercury. Which test could be used?

First, construct a summary of the available data:

Variable	Value	Level of measurement
Smoking	Cigarettes/day	Interval—not normal
Blood pressure	mm Hg	Interval—normal

Following the decision tree, we are first asked 'Are both measurements interval?'. Obviously they are, so we take the 'Y' route to the left where we are next asked, 'Are both normally distributed?' Inspection of our data has shown us that, since 60% of our sample do not smoke, the distribution curve of the number of cigarettes smoked in our sample is decidedly positively skewed. Therefore we answer 'N' on our decision tree and this leads us to the box that suggests that Spearman's rank correlation coef-

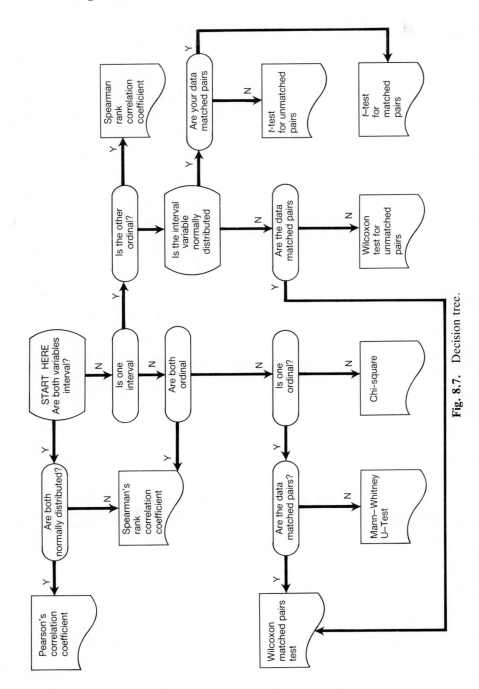

Fig. 8.7.   Decision tree.

ficient test would be the test to use at this level of measurement. As the name suggests this is a test of ·correlation and attempts to show that a change in one variable is associated with a change in the second variable. Of course there is nothing to stop us altering our level of measurement, reducing it to a lower level, for example, by simply categorizing the response to the smoking questionnaire into 'smokers' and 'non-smokers'. This would now mean that one of the variables was now at a nominal level, while the other was still interval and normally distributed. The decision tree this time would lead us to use the Student's *t*-test for unmatched pairs.

So why use Spearman's rather than the *t*-test? It is all a matter of the amount of information we hope to obtain from the data we have collected. Knowing that the more one smokes then the more likely one's BP is to be higher, says more than just knowing that if you smoke you are more likely to have a raised BP. By and large, the higher the level of measurement you use, the more 'sensitive' is the statistical test you can employ, and therefore the more likely you can start to say something about the nature of a relationship.

In the above example you could have gone one stage further down the level of measurement path and, for example, categorized the sample into those with BPs over 150 as 'high BP' and those below 151 as 'low BP'. Your two variables would now be at the lowest level of measurement, both would be nominal. In a preliminary analysis of your data it is often worthwhile doing this. By reducing your data to dichotomous variables you can construct a 'two-by-two' table (see Chapter 7) and apply a low-level test which, from the decision tree, you will see is the Chi-square test. In this way you should get a good feel for what your data contains before applying more sophisticated statistical tests.

Exercise 8(6)

In the Norman Project, what tests could be employed to examine the following null hypotheses?

(a) The level of exercise undertaken by men is not associated with socio-economic status.
(b) Being overweight is not associated with perceived stress.
(c) Non-smokers do not exercise more than smokers.
(d) Smoking behaviour is unrelated to gender.

Suggested answers are given at the end of the chapter.

SOME COMMON TESTS OF SIGNIFICANCE

Chi-square

This is a very commonly used test of association. It can be used with any level of measurement, but does require there to be a very limited number of categories of results, e.g. owner-occupier or tenant against income less than £20 000/year or £20 000 or more per year. A typical case would be results which can be included in a 2 × 2 or 2 × 3 table. The basis of the test relies on calculating what the expected number of one variable should be if it was associated with the other by chance, and then comparing this with the observed result.

Question 8(8)

Is self-perception of stress higher in women?

We would initially rephrase this in the form of the null hypothesis: there is not a higher level of stress felt by women than by men.

From Norman's results we know that 24 (48%) of the men admitted to a stress score of more than 1, while 35 (70%) of the women did so. Is this difference real or an artefact of the sampling? For the whole group of 100 men and women, 59 (24 + 35) admitted to some degree of stress. Therefore by chance we could have expected 59/100 of the 50 men and 59/100 of the 50 women to admit to some stress. We can show these *expected* results along with the *observed* results in Table 8.9.

Table 8.9.

	Stress <2		Stress >1	
	Expected	Observed	Expected	Observed
Men	21.5	26	29.5	24
Women	21.5	15	29.5	35

There does appear to be a difference. Fewer men and more women admit to some level of stress than one would expect. Is the result significant? To find out we use the Chi-square test.

The difference between the expected and the observed result is calculated for each of the compartments in the table. This difference is then squared to remove the negative signs, divided by the expected result and these results are added together to give the Chi-square statistic.

$$\text{Chi-sq} = \frac{(21.5 - 26)^2}{21.5} + \frac{(29.5 - 24)^2}{29.5} + \frac{(21.5 - 15)^2}{21.5} + \frac{(29.5 - 35)^2}{29.5}$$
$$= 0.94 + 1.02 + 1.97 + 1.02$$
$$= 4.95$$

We now need to look up in a table of Chi-square (found at the back of most, if not all, texts on statistics) to see whether this result is to be expected. To use the table you will also need to know the *degrees of freedom* available. This is a technical issue but easily calculated. The degrees of freedom in a table equals the sum of the number of columns in a table minus 1, times the number of rows in a table minus 1. In the example above, a two-by-two table, i.e. two columns by two rows, this means the number of degrees of freedom is $(2-1) \times (2-1)$, that is there is 1 degree of freedom for this table. In the table of Chi-square you will find that for 1 degree of freedom a Chi-square of 4.95 would be found on fewer than 1 in 20 ($p<0.05$) occasions. It is therefore unlikely that the result was a 'fluke' and so we can safely reject the null hypothesis. Women in this study report more stress and this is *statistically significant*.

Exercise 8(7)

Do people who exercise regularly (i.e. exercise score more than 1) feel less stressed?

Suggested answers are given at the end of the chapter.

In summary, Chi-square can be used to show an *association* between variables whatever the level of measurement, as long as the number of categories for both variables is limited. It must also be remembered that Chi-squared measures the significance of the association between variables, but makes no judgement about the underlying strength of that association.

But what if the number of categories is not limited to a small number— how then do you draw conclusions about differences that exist between samples?

Question 8(9)

Are men in Norman's sample more likely to be overweight than the women?

The null hypothesis is that men are not more likely to be overweight than women. Tabulating our variables as before:

Variable	Value	Level of measurement
Weight	BMI	interval
Sex	Male/female	nominal

We know that the index we have chosen, the Body-Mass Index, is an interval-ratio measured unit—the highest level of measurement. Looking at the frequency-distribution charts earlier also leads us to suspect that the distribution of results does follow a normal-shaped curve. This allows us to use more sensitive tests to explore whether the null hypothesis is supported or rejected.

Our decision tree shows us that we could employ the *t*-test for unmatched pairs. The *t*-test examines how much overlap there is between the population suggested by one sample and that suggested by the second sample. Do the figures suggest that the degree of overlap is sufficiently large to assume that the two samples are from the same population and that no true difference exists?

Mann–Whitney U-test

This is a non-parametric alternative to the *t*-test for unpaired data. It can therefore be used when one of the variables has been measured at an interval level but which is not normally distributed, or for data measured at an ordinal level. The other variable is measured at a nominal level. For example, it could be sex, i.e. 'men' and 'women', against 'number of cigarettes smoked per day'. The test is performed by looking at the relative *ranking* of the two samples if they are regarded as a single population. The sum of the ranks in the smaller sample (if unequal sized samples are being compared) is calculated and this can be compared with expected values for known sample sizes by looking at the relevant tables. If the figure calculated is greater or less than expected at the 0.05 level then one can say that it is likely that the samples represent different populations.

Matched pairs

In the decision tree you will have seen that one of the questions asked is whether pairs of data are matched or not. What is meant by this? Matching is built into the design of a project to eliminate as many possible 'hidden' differences between the samples as possible. In a simple 'before and after' design, the sample subjects are compared before and after an experimental variable has been introduced. In this sense the variable measured before is 'paired' with that measured afterwards, and so can be said to be matched. Another design may employ experimental and control groups which have been paired as closely as possible for as many variables as possible other than those involved in the experiment. Again the data from the two groups could be considered to be paired or matched. If the 50 men and 50 women in the study had been selected as 50 married couples then we could have compared men and women for whatever variable we wished to look at by looking at these matched pairs. Being married would have eliminated many socio-economic and other characteristics that may otherwise unknowingly have influenced the result.

There are two tests that can be used for data from matched pairs. One is the Wilcoxon matched pairs test, which assumes in fact a level of measurement slightly higher than ordinal, but can be used for non-parametric data, and the *t*-test for paired data for normally distributed variables.

In the Wilcoxon test, the difference between the value of each of the pairs is calculated and then these differences are ranked, ignoring the sign of the difference. The sum of these ranks are calculated for the positve and negative differences. If the two samples are from the same population, there is as likely to be a negative difference as there is a positive one, and so the sum of the negative ranks should about equal the sum of the positive ranks. The smaller of these two sums can be compared from tables for the known sample size (i.e. the number of pairs), and a probability for that figure found, thereby supporting the null hypothesis that both samples came from the same population.

TESTS OF CORRELATION

It is often possible from the raw data to get the impression that as one variable changes so does another. Now if there was such a relationship, and we knew what it was, then we could be in a position to estimate one of the variables if we knew the value of the other. Correlation and regression tests will give an indication of the extent to which a change in one variable is matched by change in another. By how much will my weight increase if my height increases by 10%? How much more likely am I to contract heart disease if I smoke 60 as opposed to 10 cigarettes a day?

There are two tests commonly used to demonstrate and quantify the degree of correlation. Spearman's rank correlation coefficient for non-parametric interval data, or the product moment correlation coefficient (Pearson's) for instances when both variables being examined are interval and normally distributed.

Spearman's rank correlation coefficient

With this test the two variables are again ranked in order. If the two variables are not associated at all, then the rank of the second variable would be random and unrelated to the ranking of the first variable. On the other hand, if one of the variables was entirely dependent on the other, then the ranks would be identical. Spearman's test gives a measure of how well the ranking of the two tests agree. This measure runs from -1, which suggests that as one goes up, the other goes down unit by unit, to $+1$ where a unit increase in one corresponds to a unit increase in the other. If there is absolutely no correlation at all between the two variables, then Spearman's correlation coefficient will be zero. Again, tables provide significance levels for any correlation coefficient: if, for example, we had 10 pairs, a Spearman's correlation coefficient of 0.56 would only be significant at the 0.1 level, i.e. there is a 1 in 10 likelihood that the result could have occurred by chance. If, on the other hand, we had 30 pairs, a correlation coefficient of 0.36 is significant at the 0.05 level.

For normally distributed sets of data a corresponding correlation coefficient, Pearson's '*r*', can be calculated running from the same limits of -1 to $+1$.

Other tests

We have deliberately only looked at a small number of all the available tests which can be found in textbooks and elsewhere. Some others commonly used are:

ANOVA, or analysis of variance, which allows more than two sets of variables to be compared.

Regression, which enables one variable to be predicted by another.

Factor analysis, which, from a stew-pot bubbling with variables, tries to link together those that appear to be connected.

There are many, many tests for many occasions. We have tried to point out those most commonly and easily used.

SUMMARY

Statistics is to many a confused and confusing area. Exactly what test to use and how to carry out that test present great problems. This latter aspect, how to do the test, is nowadays much easier with the fairly wide availability of sophisticated statistics packages for microcomputers, which will not only do the test for you, but allow you to manipulate your data between levels of measurement to allow a variety of tests on the same data.

At the end of the day, you will be trying to indicate how likely it is that any differences between two variables you are comparing could have arisen by chance. In an ideal world you would have discussed your whole project with a medical statistician and geared the design of your project, including the type of question and level of data response, to answer a specific question for which a particular statistical test has been selected. This would include, in most cases, an opportunity to estimate the size of the sample required to confirm the degree of difference you are wanting to show at a pre-determined level of statistical significance. The statistics thus assume a prominent role in the design of the project. Unfortunately this is not an ideal world. Medical statisticians still need to be sought out—departments of general practice would be a start, departments of community medicine in districts another possibility. Even if this has not been done and you arrive at the stage of data analysis, there is still hope that much can be obtained from your data by careful consideration of the question, the level of measurement obtained, and the type of tests available. Go forth and multiply, or divide, add ... whatever!

SUGGESTED TASKS

1.   Carry out a one-week audit of your appointments system, establishing for each patient the gap between the time they would like to be seen
and the time they do actually get a consultation. Prepare some tables and
figures that summarize your results.

2.   Carry out a one-week audit of all your consultations, noting
whether your patients are male or female. Ask a colleague (possibly one of
the opposite sex) to do likewise and compare your results using the
Chi-square test.

ANSWERS TO EXERCISES

Exercise 8(1)

(a)   We would suggest a pie-chart.

(b)   and (c)   We would suggest bar-charts.

Exercise 8(2)

The mean BMI for the men was 24.56, and for the women 23.02.
How did you calculate the sum of the BMIs? Did you add together all
the individual scores, or did you take advantage of the work you had
already done in categorizing the results? Using the latter, the sum of all the
BMIs would have been:

$$(20 \times 4) + (21 \times 2) + (22 \times 2) + (23 \times 8) + (24 \times 6) + (25 \times 15)$$
$$+ (26 \times 5) + (27 \times 2) + (28 \times 2) + (29 \times 2) + (30) + (31).$$

Always try to take the easiest route, and avoid duplicating work.

Exercise 8(3)

(a)   The median value for the men was 125, compared with a mean of
126.9. The median for the women was also 125 compared with a mean of
126.1.

(b)   The median BMI for the men was 25, with mean 24.6; and for the
women the median was 22.5, with mean 23.0.

For all these results there is fairly close agreement between the mean
and median figures, suggesting that there is a degree of regular symmetry
about the distribution of the results.

Exercise 8(4)

The mean BMI for the men was 24.6 with a SD of 2.5. For the women the SD was 3.3 around a mean of 23.0.

Exercise 8(5)

The SE for the men was 0.4, and for the women the SE was 0.5.

The mean BMI for the men aged 35 to 40 in the practice is between 23.8 and 25.4 at the 95% confidence level. For the women the mean BMI is between 22.0 and 24.0 at the 95% confidence level.

Exercise 8(6)

(a)   Level of exercise is ordinal, as is social class. Following the decision tree leads one to Spearman's rank correlation coefficient.

(b)   Weight (BMI) is interval and normally distributed. Stress is ordinal. Again, the decision tree suggests that Spearman's is the test to employ.

(c)   Smoking is nominal in this study, and exercise ordinal. The decision tree suggests that the Mann–Whitney U-test could be tried.

(d)   Smoking and gender are both nominal. Chi-squared is the test suggested.

Exercise 8(7)

The null hypothesis is: People who exercise do not have a lower degree of perceived stress.

The frequency table looks like

	Stress <2		Stress >1	
	Expected	Observed	Expected	Observed
Exercise	19.3	23	27.7	24
No exercise	21.7	17	31.3	36

Chi-squared = 2.92. The degrees of freedom number 3. Tables of Chi-squared show that this is not significant at the 0.05 level and so the null hypothesis is supported.

9 Writing up the research

The chapters so far have described in detail the various stages of the research process, beginning with defining a question for research and developing a research design, through to analysing the data collected in the study using a range of statistical techniques. This chapter focuses on describing the various questions and issues that need to be tackled when writing up the research.

Dr Greatman has been investigating the relationship between the allocation of time in general practice and list size. He has carried out a survey of a random sample of 200 general practitioners working in the Region. Fifty five per cent of the general practitioners completed and sent back his mail questionnaire, giving an achieved sample of 110. These data have been coded and put on the computer. His analysis has shown that list size is modestly but positively correlated to both hours worked per week in surgery consultations and hours worked per week in all work-related activities. However, list size is inversely but once again only modestly associated with consultation rates, home visiting rates, and consultation length.

Dr Greatman thinks that his findings are important and interesting but how does he tell other people about them? He phones his golfing colleague, a partner at a local Health Centre, to give him the exciting news. His colleague mumbles 'Oh, how interesting' and rather deflatedly Dr Greatman puts down the phone. He could, on the other hand, give a talk to colleagues, but must he wait in hope for the invitation that never comes? Anyway this would only reach a small number of people. He decides that the only answer is to write up the results for publication in an academic journal; that way he will reach a wide audience and maybe achieve just a little bit of fame.

WHAT SORT OF DOCUMENT?

There are two options:

(a) a report which contains a detailed account of the study and analysis of findings;

(b) a paper or article for publication.

Reports are detailed descriptions of the study as a whole and tend to be required by grant-giving bodies to show what was finally produced with their money. However, the distribution of such a report is likely to be limited and it will probably be too long and detailed for people to read in any depth. It is therefore more usual to try for a publication, not just to be seen as clever and famous but because it obtains the widest possible readership. There are, in addition, other advantages of publication:

- Publication in a reputable journal using scientific referees implies that the research is of good quality.
- Publication is crucial in the development of a research career, and without publication it is increasingly difficult to make progress and gain further financial support.

Dr Greatman is aware that his paper might not be accepted for publication and he might end up with nothing to show for his painstaking efforts. However, he is also aware of the proliferation of new journals in the area and as a last resort feels—somewhat arrogantly—that he can always 'dump' his paper in one of the possibly less prestigious journals.

HOW SHOULD A SCIENTIFIC PAPER BE STRUCTURED?

The most common structure for a paper involves it being divided up into four sections:

(a) Introduction;
(b) Methods;
(c) Results;
(d) Discussion (and conclusion).

WRITING THE INTRODUCTORY SECTION

The introduction sets the scene for the study. It should include a brief review of the main literature in the area, citing and summarizing important earlier studies. This should be followed by a statement of the question that the research has tried to answer. The skill in writing the literature review is to get it to the point where the research question seems the next natural step. Alternatively, especially when there is little existing literature, a few sentences may be necessary to justify and explain the importance of the study.

Dr Greatman sits down that weekend after a visit to the library to write the first draft of his intended introductory section:

Draft: Smith[1] found little evidence of any variation with list size in the total number of hours spent each week by general practitioners in patient care. Jones and Marsh[2] found a similar pattern of evidence to Smith as did White[3]. Wilcalfe and Metkin[4] found a strong positive correlation between list size and the aggregate amount of time spent each week in surgery consultations and home visits. Swift[5] found little evidence of an association between list size and consultation rate and home visiting rate although the opposite pattern was found by Davis[6]. Wilcalfe and Metkin[4] found little evidence of an association between list size and consultation length.

This study further explores the relationship between list size and the allocation of time in general practice. This question is of importance because it has been argued[7] that lowering list sizes would lead to a better standard of care in general practice. This research therefore addresses one of the most important issues in general practice today and its findings should have far-reaching consequences in health policy in this area.

Q.1.   What are the major weaknesses in this introductory section?

(a)   It is better to move from the general to the specific rather than the specific to the general. Thus, the policy questions in the second paragraph about the impact of lowering list sizes on the standard of care might have been raised at the beginning of the paper, putting the more specific research question in a broader context. It might also be necessary to spell out the assumed link between reduction in list size, release of time, and improvement in the standards of care.

(b)   The introduction should describe how the research links with the pattern of evidence and the development of the research which has been published previously on the topic. Thus, it is a matter of identifying the key research in the area to show how this previously published research supports or illustrates arguments in the paper. The major problem with the introduction as it stands at present is that the research studies which are described tend to duplicate one another. Also, the literature tends to lead the argument, and the implications of the previous evidence for the current research study are not clearly drawn out.

(c)   The introduction should contain an explanation or explanations for carrying out the specific piece of work. No reasons are given in this introduction on why it is necessary to further examine the link between list size and the allocation of time. Why is this new research superior to that which has previously been carried? What are its novel qualities? Does it deal with a question previously neglected in the research, or does it attempt to overcome the methodological deficiencies inherent in previous studies?

(d)   The introduction should also contain a description of the specific objectives and propositions to be examined. No such description is found here, e.g. what is the relationship between: (i) list size and hours spent per week in patient contact and all work-related activities, (ii) consultation rate and home visiting rate, and (iii) consultation length?

(e)   The introduction should also contain a description of the general method of investigation, i.e. include a statement such as 'drawing on evidence collected from a survey carried out on a random sample of 200 GPs in a region, this study examined the association between ...'

(f)   The final sentence may reflect the researcher's pride in the work carried out, but scientific convention requires more modesty and an assumption that the reader will judge the importance of the study.

In summary, the introductory section should:

(1)   begin with a broad issue or problem and move towards a more specific research question;

(2)   identify the key research in the area and use it to illustrate the paper's arguments;

(3)   identify the novel qualities of the proposed research and give explanations for carrying out this particular project;

(4)   describe the objectives of the study and the specific proposition(s) to be explored;

(5)   describe the general method of investigation;

(6)   not claim too much for the work.

Here is a rewritten version of the introduction which attempts to incorporate each of these points.

For several years the policy of the General Medical Services Committee has been that list sizes in general practice should fall to a target national average of 1700. This is usually justified on the grounds that smaller lists produce higher standards of care.[1] The key factor that is believed to mediate the relation between list sizes and standards of care is time; if general practitioners acquire smaller lists, the argument runs, they will have time to enhance the standard of care in their practices[2] through extending their consultation time.

In his review of published studies up to 1980, Butler found little evidence of any systematic variation with list size in the total number of hours spent each week by general practitioners in caring for patients[3]. The extra time available to doctors with smaller lists was much less likely to be spent on longer consultations than on higher rates of consultation in the surgery and home visiting. In their study of 199 general practitioners in inner and outer Manchester, Wilkin and Metcalfe[4] found a strong positive correlation between list size and the aggregate amount of time spent each week on consultations and home visits. This study did, however, support the earlier work[5] in showing that there is no more than a slight relation between list size and length of consultation and an inverse association between list size and the rate of consultation. Thus, it may be unrealistic to expect general practitioners to respond automatically to smaller lists by increasing their length of consultations.

There are, however, deficiencies in previous studies; they were often confined to self-selected practitioners, sometimes had low rates of response, and did not usually measure the allocation of time among all the components of the working week. In this study an attempt was made to surmount these deficiencies and a survey was carried out based on a random sample of GPs working in the Region. The objective of the study was to investigate to what extent list size influences the amount of time a GP spends in work-related activities.

WRITING THE METHODS SECTION

The methods section should present the method used with sufficient clarity and detail, such that the reader would be able to replicate the study.

Now, satisfied with the introduction, Dr Greatman drafts out the next section:

Draft: The data collected in this study were derived from information gathered from 110 general practitioners working in the Region. This information included data on personal list size, on booking interval, on consultation rate and home visiting rate, and hours worked per week on a range of work-related activities. An analysis was carried out examining the relationship between personal list size and the indices of time.

Q.2.   What are the weaknesses of the methods section?

(a)   There is a complete absence of information about the research design and why a cross-sectional survey was used to test the specific proposition.

(b)   No information was given about the sampling frame, the sample size, or the method of sampling. In the study a 55% response rate was achieved, which is quite low, so it will be necessary to show that the responders do not differ in any significant way from the non-responders. If they do differ, it is important to show if and how they may influence the interpretation of the results.

(c)   There is also an absence of information about the method of data collection. A mail questionnaire was chosen, with a reminder postcard three weeks later, followed by a reminder letter three weeks after the postcard. Any pilot studies also need to be described.

(d)   There is also an absence of information about why the concepts were operationalized in the way they were. Why was personal list size chosen as the definition of list size? How were the consultation rate and home visiting rate calculated and why was booking interval used as an indicator of consultation length?

(e)   There needs to be at least some assessment of the reliability and validity of the measures used in the study. Doctors' own descriptions of hours worked per week on work-related activities were used and there needs to be some indication that these measures based on self-report and retrospective information do not suffer from any major biases. If there are biases, then it is important to explain how they might influence the interpretation of the results. One way of assessing reliability is by comparing the findings with those from studies using different methodologies.

(f)   There is an absence of information about the form of the analysis. What statistical tests were going to be used and why?

In summary, the methods section should contain:

(1)   descriptions of sampling frame, sampling method, sample size, response rate, representativeness of the responders, and explanation for the methodology chosen;

(2)   description of the method of data collection and how the instrument was piloted;

(3)   discussion and explanation of how and why the concepts were operationalized in the way they were;

(4)   assessment of the reliability and validity of the instrument;

(5)   description of techniques to be used in the analyses.

Here is a revised version of the methods section which attempts to incorporate each of these points.

The study was a postal survey of unrestricted principals in the Region. The addresses of the 200 doctors selected were obtained from the FPC lists. The first mailing was sent in October 1984, and two follow-up mailings were used. Altogether 110 doctors replied, giving a response rate of 55%.

Seven characteristics were obtained for most of the non-responders as well as the responders: year and place of qualification, sex, whether they were members of the RCGP, personal list size, average list size in the practice, and geographical location. No significant differences between responders and non-responders was found for any of the characteristics, suggesting that there were not any serious biases in the response.

All the data were collected through a self-completed questionnaire and the questions had been piloted in a small study of trainers ($n = 20$). All the information collected was based on doctors' reports and was not validated from independent sources. However, it appears this reliance on self-reported information, with the possible problems of biases in reporting, may not be of particular importance judging from comparisons with similar data gathered from other studies which used different methodologies. For example, a recent national study of GP workload[5] using diaries as their method of data collection reported that, on average, general practitioners spend 38 hours a week on General Medical Services (GMS) and six hours on the non-General Medical Service activities. The figures for GMS and non-GMS activities found in this study were 37.2 and 4.3 hours respectively.

In addition to the indices of time, another key variable in the analyses is list size, and it can be calculated in a number of different ways. The primary focus of the study was on the performance of individual GPs and so it was decided to collect information about the personal lists of the respondents in the survey. The statistical relationship between personal list size and the allocation of time was analysed using Pearson's correlation coefficient.

WRITING THE RESULTS SECTION

The results section is where the findings are presented. The commonest failing here is to give too many results in too much detail. Remember that the reader does not have either the same intimate knowledge or interest in every detail. Try to summarize. As an incentive many journals restrict the number of tables permitted to about six.

Dr Greatman writes the draft of his results section:

Draft: Table 9.1 shows the distribution of the estimates of time spent per week in a range of practice-based activities. The table shows marked variations in time spent on both surgery consultations and home visits which were the activities which made up the bulk of the working week for most doctors.

Table 9.2 shows the strength of the relationship between list size and the indices of time. The table shows that list size was negatively associated with booking interval, consultation rate, and home visiting rate but positively correlated with numbers of hours in surgery consultations and all practice-based activities.

Q.3.   What are the major weaknesses in the results section?

(a)   Table 9.1 contains a large amount of information and it would be much clearer if the table was broken down into practice-based activities and activities outside the practice, e.g. private practice, etc.

(b)   Table 9.1 contains figures which are percentages rather than actual values and yet there is no mention of percentages in the table. Also there is no information on sample size for each of the categories.

(c)   Table 9.2 presents a correlation matrix but there was no reference

Table 9.1. *Estimates of time spent each week on all activities*

	None	1	–2	–3	–4	>4	≤5	10	15	20	25	30	>30	Mean number of hours
Surgery consultations	—	—	—	—	—	—	1	3	19	41	—	10	5	20
Home visits	—	—	—	—	—	—	20	45	22	10	3	1	1	10.5
Practice administration	—	—	—	—	—	—	85	13	2	1	1	—	—	3.2
Reading, research	—	—	—	—	—	—	87	11	2	1	1	1	—	2.9
Training courses	—	—	—	—	—	—	—	—	—	—	—	—	—	
Other	—	—	—	—	—	—	88	10	1	1	—	—	—	2.2
Private practice	83	10	3	1	1	2	—	—	—	—	—	—	—	0.4
Hospital appointment	70	2	4	4	6	13	—	—	—	—	—	—	—	
Insurance work	48	34	13	4	2	1	—	—	—	—	—	—	—	0.7
Clinic	77	6	10	3	2	2	—	—	—	—	—	—	—	0.6
Police and industrial work	84	6	4	1	2	3	—	—	—	—	—	—	—	0.5
Committee work	78	12	5	2	1	2	—	—	—	—	—	—	—	0.4
Teaching	91	5	2	1	1	1	—	—	—	—	—	—	—	0.2
Other	86	3	3	2	1	4	—	—	—	—	—	—	—	0.4

Table 9.2. *Interrelationships between list size and indices of time*

	List size	Booking interval	No of hours in surgery consultations	No. of hours in all activities	Consultation rate	Home visiting rate
List size	—					
Booking interval	−0.1941	—				
No. of hours in surgery consultation	0.2570	0.13638	—			
No. of hours in all activities	0.2034	0.06323	0.58919	—		
Consultation rate	−0.33842	−0.09077	0.12527	0.12046	—	
Home visiting rate	−0.2004	−0.07448	0.01742	0.19420	0.19920	—

to the specific statistical correlation test being used nor were there any details of levels of statistical significance.

(d)   Although the strength of the interrelationships between the indices of time is of interest, it is not directly relevant to this particular analysis. The aim here is to examine the strength of the relationship between list size and the indices of time. While the correlation is useful, it might have been better to present these relationships in the form of graphs.

(e)   Some of the correlations were to five decimal places and others to four. It is better to have consistency throughout and four decimal places are probably sufficient.

In summary, the results section should contain:

(1)   clear tables or graphs which do not contain too much information or irrelevant information;

(2)   a clear and concise commentary on the tables and graphs highlighting the major points;

(3)   information about sample sizes, statistical tests used, and levels of statistical significance should also be presented;

(4)   graphs and figures are sometimes clearer ways of illustrating the strength and nature of relationships between variables.

Examples of how the data could be presented are shown in the following tables and graphs. Tables 9.3 and 9.4 illustrate how to present the data about doctors' estimates of time spent on practice-based activities (Table 9.3) and non-practice-based activities (Table 9.4). The tables include both values and percentages and sample sizes for each activity. Figure 9.1 illustrates how data can be presented in the form of a graph. It shows the relationship between personal list size and number of hours worked per week and gives a much clearer picture than just presenting correlations or tables.

WRITING THE DISCUSSION

The discussion section is where inferences from the findings are drawn and where conclusions are presented. There is often a tendency to put results in the discussion and vice versa. Try to keep them separate.

At last a break in a busy morning for Dr Greatman; the Placebo Pharmaceutical's representative has phoned to say his car has broken down: time for Dr Greatman to set out the discussion:

Draft: The results from this study clearly show that list size is strongly related to the time general practitioners spend at work. The results showed that as list size decreased the doctors spent less time at work

Table 9.3. *Respondents' estimates of the time spent each week on GMS activities*

| | Distribution of respondents' estimates | | | | | | | | |
Hours per week spent on:	5 hours or less (%)	5.1 to 10.0 hours (%)	10.1 to 15.0 hours (%)	15.1 to 20.0 hours (%)	20.1 to 30.0 hours (%)	25.1 to 30. hours (%)	more than 30 hours (%)	n (=100%)	Mean
Surgery consultations	1	3	19	41	22	10	5	1390	20.0
Home visits (including travelling)	20	45	22	10	3	1	—	1378	10.5
Practice administration	85	13	2	—	—	—	—	1410	3.2
Reading, research, training courses	87	11	2	1	—	—	—	1409	2.9
Other	88	10	1	1	—	—	—	1411	2.2
All GMS activities									38.8

Table 9.4.   *Respondents' estimates of the time spent each week on non-GMS activities*

		Distribution of respondents' estimates					
	None (%)	1 hour or less (%)	1.1 to 2.0 hours (%)	2.1 to 3.0 hours (%)	3.1 to 4.00 hours (%)	more than 4 hours (%)	n (=100%)	Mean
Hours per week spent on:								
Private practice	83	10	3	1	—	2	1413	0.4
Hospital appointments	70	2	4	4	6	13	1399	1.4
Insurance work	48	34	13	4	2	—	1377	0.7
Clinics	77	6	10	3	2	2	1406	0.6
Police/industrial work	84	6	4	1	2	3	1347	0.5
Committee work	78	12	5	2	1	2	1391	0.4
Teaching	91	5	2	1	1	1	1385	0.2
Other	86	3	3	2	1	4	1394	0.5
All non-GMS activities								4.7

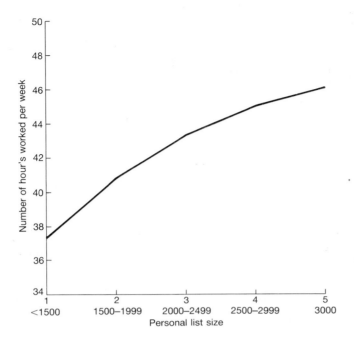

Fig. 9.1. Relationship between number of hours worked and personal list size.

overall but increased their rate of consultation and rate of home visiting and increased the length of their consultation. These findings provide strong support for those who wish to see further reductions in list size. There is clear evidence from this study that a fall in list size will lead to doctors reinvesting the extra time released into improving existing care and developing new forms of care. Thus, future policy might concentrate on moving towards the General Medical Services Committee's target of a national average list size of 1700, as this evidence suggests the pay-off would be a large one.

Q.4   What are the major weaknesses in this discussion section?

(a)   The discussion and conclusions drawn from the study do not reflect the pattern of results which were actually found. The strength of the relationship between list size and any of the indices was never more than modest, and in the case of home visiting rates was quite weak. Thus, the implication that list size was strongly associated with at least some of the indices of time is not entirely accurate.

(b)   The research design used was a cross-sectional one and the study investigated the relationship between variables. It is not possible using this kind of design to tell in which direction the causal relationship goes. Does list size determine hours spent in patient care or vice versa? To examine this question, a longitudinal design would be necessary to find support for the conclusion that a reduction in list size would lead to a fall in hours worked and increase in consultation rate, home visiting rate, and consultation length. Maybe a study using a longitudinal design should be a recommendation for further research. This type of recommendation usually comes in the final paragraph of the discussion.

In summary, the discussion section should:

(1)   Contain a broad discussion of the findings which should include explanations for ambiguous or apparently contradictory findings.

(2)   Contain the various possible interpretations of the relationship between variables.

(3)   Show how far the findings are similar to or different from those found in other research projects.

(4)   Conclude with a statement of what the study has shown and, if appropriate, suggested directions for future research in this area.

Here is an example of how a revised version of the discussion, which attempts to incorporate each of these points, might look.

It has been argued that for GPs to be able to provide new forms of care or improve existing care they need additional resources, including time. Extra time can be created through further reductions in list size. Evidence from this study provided only partial support for this argument. The evidence suggested that personal list size was particularly important for explaining variations in hours spent in surgery consultation and surgery consultation rates. This finding corroborates evidence from other studies,[3] although Wilkins and Metcalfe[4] found that the pattern was not consistent over the full range of list sizes.

The weakest relationship between the indices of time and list size was with consultation length. While there was a statistically significant trend, it was not a strong one and this is consistent with other studies which have also shown the lack of any systematic association between list sizes, and average face-to-face contacts.[6]

In conclusion, the evidence from this study suggests that while list size may be a key enabling factor in creating the conditions which give the general practitioners more time to spend, possibly in patient care or other work-related activities, it still does not fully account for variations in the allocation of time amongst these activities. The implications of these findings for policy suggest that the relationship between list sizes and doctors' behaviour is more complicated than is generally implied in the arguments about the beneficial effects of reducing the national average list size. Certainly, the evidence suggests that other changes are also required for doctors to change their behaviour and reinvest the time released from lower surgery hours into spending longer consultations with their patients.

COMPLETING THE MANUSCRIPT

The manuscript is almost complete but needs some additional information.

1.   The beginning of the paper needs to have a *title page* and an *abstract* or *summary*. The title page should contain the title of the paper, the names and qualifications of the authors, and the addresses of the authors, particularly for correspondence.

The abstract, or summary, is an important section, which in some ways is the most difficult to write. It is important because it is sometimes the only section that is read by those browsing through the journal. The aim is to write a clear précis of why the work was done, how it was done, what the findings were, and what the findings mean.

2.   The end of the text may require an *acknowledgements* paragraph, listing people who have made a significant contribution to the study, e.g. interviewers, secretaries, clerical assistants, advisers, and consultants. They should be acknowledged along with others who have made detailed and constructive comments on the paper. Financial sponsors should also be acknowledged.

3.   The text finishes with a list of *references*. This can be one of the most irritating and annoying aspects of preparing a paper for publication. One of the problems is ensuring that you have the full references for all the literature that you wish to cite. If you do not adopt the practice of writing the references out in full when you have identified them, then there is always the problem of remembering where you saw the paper, etc. One way around this is to have a set of index cards which you shuffle around as you wish. Another problem is *layout of references*. Every journal appears to have a different method, although there is increasing standardization. Two different approaches tend to be adopted for the citing of references in the text. First, there is the Harvard system where authors' surnames and date of publication are put in the text in brackets. Secondly, there is the use of superscript numbers, and there are two variations of this. The numbers may run sequentially through the text or be keyed to the list of references which is arranged in alphabetical order. The listing of references can, for both the Harvard system and the superscript number, be in alphabetical order but, as with the *British Medical Journal*, might be listed in superscript number order. The layout and arrangement of the references in the list at the end of the paper may also vary, and it is best to consult the

journal before writing the references down. It is important that the layout of the references complies with the journal style as, if it does not, it can unnecessarily irritate editors and delay publication. Some journals include the guidelines for the format of papers in every edition and others only include them in one or two editions throughout the year.

4.   The paper finishes with tables and figures, which should be presented on separate pages at the end of the paper, although their position in the text should be shown, for example by a blank space in which is written: 'Table ABC about here.' (This is to help the printer lay out the page in an attractive way.)

REVISING THE DRAFT

Seldom are writers able to produce the final polished version of their paper at the first attempt. It is always better, even before sending it to co-authors or colleagues, to wait a week or so and then go back to revise and rewrite those parts that are unclear. At this stage it will be possible to check the structure and accuracy of the paper. When completed, it is useful to circulate the paper for comments from friendly colleagues and to obtain agreement from persons quoted, collaborators, and sponsors. When the comments have all arrived it is time to redraft, incorporating constructive criticisms. Once this is done the paper can be retyped and shown to co-authors. When everybody agrees that it is suitable it can be sent for publication.

GETTING PUBLISHED

On receipt of a manuscript the editor of the appointed journal will send an acknowledgement and send the paper off to scientific referees, experts in the field who are invited to read and comment on the suitability of papers for publication in that particular journal. This task is an unpaid one and sometimes experts in the field feel that they have neither the time nor inclination to referee all papers sent to them: editors therefore sometimes have to try one or two experts before they find someone who will agree to take on the task. The number of referees per paper varies from journal to journal, although it is seldom more than two. The referees chosen are usually those who have expertise in the particular topic or in the methods and techniques used, and editors usually try to select referees so that they can receive a balanced interpretation of the paper. Thus, if it covers medical and social aspects, the editor may use a medical practitioner and a sociologist as referees, or if it is medical and statistical, a doctor and a statistician will be used.

Depending on the journal, referees might or might not be told the author's name(s). Authors are never told the referees' names, although sometimes they can be guessed. In addition to giving comments about originality, technical quality, clarity of presentation, and applicability to the area of the journal's interests, editors invite referees to rate the manuscript in terms of whether it should be published. These ratings tend to fall into four categories:

(1)   accept without change,

(2)   accept with minor changes,

(3)   accept only with major revision,

(4)   reject.

The editor, on receipt of all the referees' comments, will make a decision and send his or her verdict to the author, usually with either the full comments or extracts of referees' comments.

THE POLITICS OF PUBLICATION

It must be remembered that the process of gaining publication has a 'political' side to it, which will soon be apparent when you get on board the publication ego trip. Here are a few pointers for when you are thinking about submitting your paper for publication.

The idea that journals are open and impartial in their judgements about what constitutes good research is not entirely true. If you are keen to get your paper published in a specific journal, it might be sensible to have a look through the journal to see the type of article which it favours. Some journals do not like qualitative research and those which are house-journals for professional groups tend to favour papers that do not criticize the policy of those professional associations.

In some cases the author faces a dilemma. Do you submit your paper to the more conventional journal and water down the arguments for fear of rejection? Alternatively, do you leave the paper as you want it and submit to a journal with more radical views. The problem with the latter approach is that you are preaching to the converted. However, the process of gaining publication is usually a matter of negotiation between the authors, the editor, and the referees. In the end, it is important to be flexible and for authors to accept at least some criticisms and agree to some modifications.

If you are writing in an area where only one or two well-known authors have worked before, it might be possible to predict who the reviewers will be. It might be possible to prepare in advance for the criticisms and try to incorporate defences in the paper. Some authors try to overcome possible adverse reviews by sending their papers around to other researchers before submission for publication. The aim is to take account of adverse criticisms before they are officially recorded. The obvious drawback is that having seen the paper in advance the reviewer may not feel it would be fair to review it and would advise the editor accordingly if asked to comment on it.

Publication has many idiosyncratic aspects to it, although good quality work, as might be expected, has the greatest chance of publication. However, the rule of thumb is to think carefully about the most appropriate form of publication for your work. Many journals take at least three months to make a decision about publication, so choosing an inappropriate journal can waste a considerable amount of time and effort. It must also be remembered that the timelag between acceptance and appearing in print is seldom less than six months.

It is unusual for papers to be accepted at first submission. Referees and/ or editors usually want some changes, even if only grammatical. There is, of course, initial disappointment that the paper was not accepted as it stood. But, as if to rub salt into the wound, the referees' comments often seem trivial or irrelevant. No doubt they sometimes are, but they always seem particularly carping the day you receive them. Read them a couple of days later and often you begin to wonder again if perhaps referees are human after all. Remember that refereeing papers, while it confers some power, is an unpaid, unacknowledged (because it is done anonymously), and time-consuming job, and that if someone has critically analysed your paper and written a page or two of comments they deserve some appreciation.

You will be advised of any changes required in a letter from the editor, which usually contains extracts of referees' comments to aid you in revision. If the editor's/referees' advice for change is very specific then, if you want publication, you swallow hard (it might be a favourite graph or sentence that has to go) and do it. Often, however, the advice is more vague: 'shorten the paper', 'sharpen up the discussion', etc. In these circumstances you try your best to achieve these goals and resubmit the paper. Depending on the extent of changes required, the editor might or might not send the paper out again to the original referees to check whether you have made the specified changes. You might be able to influence this process if you include in your resubmitted paper a letter setting out point by point what you have changed in the original paper: a busy editor might accept your paper on the basis of this clear overview of what you have done, without paying too much heed to the actual details.

What happens if your paper is rejected? Don't despair. Carefully read the reasons given for rejection and in the light of these comments consider whether you should try another journal. There are a number of journals that accept material on research into general practice. Try each of the journals in turn (you will at least build up an interesting—and often diverse—collection of referees' comments). Then think about the GP 'comics': they need a regular flow of material, and while they don't count as 'proper' academic publications (the mark of the latter is the expert refereeing process) they will pay you for your writing. The final alternative is to write your study up as a report and circulate it to colleagues.

Exercise 9(1).

Identify the most appropriate journal(s) for publication of papers on the following topics:

(a) a survey of patient satisfaction with the health service;
(b) an audit of preventive practices in three general practices;
(c) the prevalence of hypertension in a rural population;
(d) an evaluation of a health promotion facilitator in general practice;
(e) assessing methods of treating diabetes.

suggested answers are given at the end of the chapter.

AUTHORSHIP

One of the most tricky aspects of publication is deciding on authorship. Obviously, this is not a problem if you do not have collaborators and you are the sole author. However, if others are involved, how do you decide who should or should not be co-authors and who should be the senior author (first author) who has the honour of always being cited (e.g. Einstein *et al.*). There are many 'grey' areas to this issue but the convention for allocation of the authorship status seems to be based on the nature of the contribution made by each participant. Those carrying out routine tasks, such as coding, might be acknowledged at the end of the paper. However, those who have contributed significantly in the form of ideas and creative thinking should be included as co-authors. The ordering of the authorship will depend upon the relative contribution made by each author. The person who makes the most contribution should be the first author (and that person, to earn their reward, usually writes the first draft, and co-authors then provide constructive comments and criticism). If the contributions are of equal proportion then the authorship is usually in alphabetical order.

SUMMARY

This chapter has concentrated on the writing up of the research. It has focused on issues and problems in writing a paper for publication and described the process of getting a paper published.

SUGGESTED TASKS

Read some journals. This time don't just read the abstract but note how authors have crafted their paper. Try to think critically: if you were asked to be the referee for a particular published paper, what would you have written as advice to the author? (You are able to do this because papers, in a sense, are never finished and, even if published, they could always have been further improved.)

ANSWERS TO EXERCISES

Exercise 9(1)

Suggested journals—there are no doubt more.
- (a)   *Health and Social Services Journal*; *Community Medicine*.
- (b)   *Journal of the Royal College of General Practitioners (JRCGP)*; *Journal of Family Practice*.
- (c)   *JRCGP*; *Epidemiology and Community Health*; *Community Medicine*.
- (d)   *JRCGP*; *Health Education Journal*; *Journal of Family Practice*.
- (e)   *British Medical Journal*; *Lancet*.

10 Planning research

RESEARCH PROTOCOLS

If you have not already started, now is the time to think about doing your own research. The previous chapters have covered a number of different skills you may require, although in the first instance you might like to start with something fairly straightforward, such as an audit of your workload. Then, when you see that research is not something restricted to ivory towers, you can be more ambitious.

For any research you do, even the most elementary, it is wise to prepare a statement about what you intend to do and how. This is more formally known as a *research protocol*. For a simple study it need be no longer than a page; it would start with a single sentence statement of the aim of the study and be followed by a paragraph or two on the precise method that will be used to achieve the aim. For a relatively straightforward study, such as establishing your prescribing rate over one week, it may seem that even this effort is unnecessary; however, it is a good discipline to get into and you will find that even with an uncomplicated study there will be times when a 'plan' is invaluable. In addition, putting things on to paper before you start can be very useful in identifying problems with the research. It is all too easy to sit in an armchair and imagine that the planned research is straightforward. Putting it on paper enables you to see if you have an answerable question and a viable method. Written plans enable you to show them to other people to get their comments and advice. This latter procedure is very important in working up any research proposal. A fresh eye, a different view, so often identifies silly errors or impractical plans, for even the most experienced researcher. Show your protocol to a partner, a spouse, a receptionist, etc. and ask them if it seems coherent and reasonable.

Exercise 10(1)

Write a protocol to establish your referral rate over a one-month period.

Suggested answer is given at the end of the chapter.

For research which is other than fairly basic you will need a more elaborate protocol. This will have various sections:

- Title page;
- Introduction;
- Aims;
- Methods;

- Analysis;
- Funding requirements;
- Timetable;
- References.

The first four sections are very similar to the initial sections of the research write-up described in the previous chapter.

First, there will be a *title page* with the name of the study, names of the researchers, and an address for correspondence.

Next there is the *introduction*, which sets the scene and summarizes relevant literature. *References* for the literature would be placed at the very back of the protocol. Then follows a brief but important statement of the *aims* of the study, together with any specific research question(s) that you intend to answer.

This is followed by details of the *method* you propose to use, specifically details of the overall design and sample. There is no need at this stage to include particular measurement schedules, such as questionnaires: it is only necessary to say what form of data collection will be carried out. Details of the method are followed by a very brief overview of what you intend to do in the *analysis*. Of course, very often you will not know exactly what you are going to do until you have designed your schedules and collected and coded the data, so all you can be expected to provide is an outline of which variables you are going to relate to which.

Have you completed these sections adequately? The crucial thing to look for is the coherence of the aim, method, and analysis. The method, together with the analysis, should enable you to answer the questions advanced in the aims section. It is all too easy to add in an extra lump of analysis 'because you happen to be collecting those bits of data': but if the analysis (or method) will help you to answer questions which are not posed in the aims section that does not mean you have a 'bonus' but that either the aims, methods, and/or analysis sections need rewriting. The commonest mistakes in the early days of trying to write a protocol are that the method section will answer a different question to the one set out in the aims section, and that the analysis will answer yet another. Read each of these sections carefully and ask whether they present a consistent picture.

Remember that the work you put in on these sections—perhaps several drafts as the ideas are pushed into shape—will be very useful later when you come to write up the research.

If your research plans are quite elaborate, you may need to prepare costings so as to get an overview of your *funding requirements*. Costings divide into several sections:

Labour: You will presumably work on the study yourself. Will this be 'spare' time or will it involve you in giving up clinical work and incurring locum costs? Will you need help with:

clerical work;
secretarial;
interviewing;
transcribing;
coding;
computing?

Equipment:

stationery;
stamps;
photocopying;
telephone;
tape recorder;
printing;
computer.

Miscellaneous:

travel;
conferences.

All these costs should be carefully itemized even if you hope it can be funded out of petty cash. Grant-giving bodies will expect the costs to be realistic.

The next page should be a rough breakdown of the *timetable* for the research. These are always difficult to calculate with any certainty, but the dates you do choose can act as a useful guide when you are in the middle of a project. Very roughly, research time can be divided into thirds: one-third for planning and getting ready (up to and including Chapter 4), one-third is for the actual data collection (Chaper 5), and the rest is for data analysis and writing up (Chapters 6–9). The actual details of a timetable are usually in months, e.g. pilot study, March; data collection, April–July; analysis, August–October; etc.

The final section contains the *references* from the introductory literature review.

RESEARCH FUNDING

Various sources of funding for research are available. Which one you approach will depend on the nature of your proposed study and your funding requirements. If it is a small-scale study, with local relevance, and you need help with postage, stationery, etc., then you might consider approaching local bodies with immediate concerns for health service delivery. Local Medical Committees, Family Practioner Committees, and District Health Authorities may be willing to offer you small amounts to enable you to complete a piece of research which would have implications for local health care delivery.

If your research requires additional staffing, for example a research assistant or clerical officer, then this requires considerably more money. For this you are more likely to apply to a specific grant-giving body. The particular ones you might bear in mind are:

- The Royal College of General Practitioners Research Committee, which gives out several thousand pounds every year for research in general practice.
- the locally organized research committee, which is a regional body to give out regional funds for research within the region. Regions may have other schemes: it is worth enquiring.
- The BMA gives some research grants.
- Various charities can be approached. For example, well known for the contribution to medical research are the Nuffield and Wellcome Foundations; there are lots of others, sometimes only small, but then often overlooked. Your local postgraduate library should have one of the directories of charities which fund research.
- The Department of Health and Social Security funds research in health service delivery.
- The Medical Research Council and Economic and Social Research Council both fund research in the health area.

These various funds require different formats for the application, although most follow the usual protocol format outlined above. The precise requirements can be obtained by enquiring from the funding body itself. Your application will be sent out for referees' comments (just like a paper submitted to a journal) and on the basis of these comments the fund will make its decision. Remember that this process takes time and depends very much on the speed of the referees and how frequently the fund meets to allocate grants. Bear in mind that in many cases an informal approach to the fund can help your progress: sometimes you will be advised of subjects or areas which the fund is currently interested in funding, or you might learn of a useful way of couching your application. Sometimes fund-giving bodies will negotiate with applicants, so this is worth trying.

SUMMARY

This chapter has described how to prepare a research protocol that can act as your research map or as the basis for an application for funding.

SUGGESTED TASK

Why not start doing some research.

ANSWERS TO EXERCISES

Exercise 10(1)

Referral rate protocol

Aim: To establish my referral rate to hospital out-patients over a typical month in the practice.

Method: A referral rate requires a numerator and a denominator. The numerator will be all those patients referred to hospital out-patients during September. This will exclude patients simply sent to use hospital laboratories or those sent to A and E. The denominator will be all those patients who consult with me during surgeries and home visits.

A daily schedule will be prepared on which will be noted the age and sex of all patients consulting, together with whether or not they were referred to hospital out-patients.

The numbers of patients consulting and the number referred will be calculated from the 30 schedules collected during September. Dividing the latter by the former and multiplying by 100 will give my referral rate per 100 patients consulting.

Index